Controlling Medicaid Costs
Federalism, Competition, and Choice

**Thomas W. Grannemann
and Mark V. Pauly**

American Enterprise Institute for Public Policy Research
Washington and London

Thomas W. Grannemann is a senior economist with Mathematica Policy Research, Inc.

Mark V. Pauly is professor of health care systems and public management at the University of Pennsylvania, associate editor of the *Journal of Health Economics,* and, for the academic year 1982–1983, research fellow at the International Institute of Management in Berlin.

Yale Brozen and Jack Meyer made many helpful comments and suggestions on an early draft of this monograph. Sharon Davis assisted with data assembly and computer calculations. Felicity Skidmore reviewed the manuscript from an editorial standpoint and suggested many changes that improved its readability. Susan Klett was responsible for preparation of the manuscript.

The American Enterprise Institute would like to thank the John A. Hartford Foundation of New York City for supporting the publication of this book.

Library of Congress Cataloging in Publication Data

Grannemann, Thomas W.
    Controlling Medicaid costs.

    (AEI studies; 385)
    "October 1982."
    1. Medicaid—Costs. 2. Medicaid. I. Pauly, Mark V.,
1941–   II. Title. III. Series.
HD7102.U4G685   1983   338.4'3362104252'0973   83–9993
ISBN 0–8447–3527–2
ISBN 0–8447–3515–9 (pbk.)

Printed in the United States of America

Contents

LIST OF FIGURES

1
Introduction

Many people believe the current Medicaid program is too expensive; yet it fails to cover some low-income people most of us would like to help with their medical care costs. This statement with its apparent inconsistency probably captures much of the current frustration with the Medicaid program. Is it just wishful thinking for us to expect Medicaid to perform better at lower costs? Or is there something about the current form of the Medicaid program that has led to a less than optimal allocation of Medicaid resources—that is, something that could be corrected by restructuring the program?

In this study we take an optimistic view and argue that there are in fact ways to modify the Medicaid program that would produce better results for the dollars spent. Our approach is straightforward; in the tradition of federalism, it seeks to place administrative and financial responsibilities at the most appropriate levels of government. Unlike many recent proposals for "federalism," however, which merely amount to a reshuffling of programs from one level of authority to another, our plan calls for more fundamental changes aimed at providing the means and incentives for cost control and efficient use of resources.

Stiffening cost constraints for Medicaid are a fact of current political life. Our major theme, however, is that a leaner and in some ways better benefit package could be made available to Medicaid beneficiaries if a better system of incentives for economizing on the use of resources were implemented for governmental decision makers, providers, and beneficiaries themselves. Such a system could be devised by changing the signals to state governments to encourage them to offer a more equitable but less costly benefit package tailored to the particular characteristics of their states' Medicaid clients and medical care markets. A combination of supplementable voucher-like arrangements and greater administrative flexibility and responsibility for the states would provide the means to meet the medical care needs of the poor in a less costly and more equitable way.

The reforms proposed here are directed to the major problems of Medicaid, including rapidly growing expenditures, inequitable

1

TABLE 1

MEDICAID COSTS, 1980–1983

(billions of dollars)

Fiscal Year	Federal	State and Local	Total
1980	14.6	11.2	25.8
1981	17.1	13.3	30.4
1982	17.5	14.9	32.4
1983[a]	19.3	16.2	35.5

NOTE: Figures include vendor payments and administrative cost.

a. Estimates.

SOURCES: *Budget of the United States Government Fiscal Year 1982; Budget of the United States Government Fiscal Year 1983;* and *Budget of the United States Government Fiscal Year 1984.*

treatment of recipients, and inequitable distribution of costs among taxpayers. The Medicaid program now costs over $35 billion annually and is consuming an ever-increasing share of federal and state government budgets. The costs in recent years are shown in table 1. Federal expenditures alone are expected to rise from $18 billion in 1982 to between $24 and $26 billion by 1985. As the nation's principal program for paying the medical bills of the poor, Medicaid has been affected by the rapid increases in medical care prices generally. These increases alone, however, cannot explain the recent growth in Medicaid expenditures, which have also reflected a growth in services used per recipient. The apparent lack of control over service use by Medicaid recipients and over medical care costs in general has led the various participants in the system—state and federal governments and various groups of providers—to blame one another for inflation in Medicaid costs. But the policy debate has produced no simple solution to the Medicaid cost problem.

The prominent attention focused on the issue of costs in these public discussions has obscured other, equally serious problems of the Medicaid program. Of particular concern is the inequitable treatment of some subgroups of the poor population. While the federal government provides over half of Medicaid funds in the form of open-ended matching grants to states, state and local governments have considerable freedom to establish their own criteria for Medicaid eligibility and their own benefit levels. Thus a poor person in a state with low benefits may be ineligible for assistance, while a similarly situated person in a high-benefit state could receive virtually unlimited medical services at no charge. Categorical eligibility criteria also exclude many poor persons from benefits because of their household structure. Another concern is that Medicaid's all-or-nothing coverage creates a benefit notch that acts as a disincentive for some low-income persons to seek employment.

The current direction of federal policy on Medicaid is unclear. The rising cost of the program has provoked a strong desire by policy makers to control, limit, or cap its rate of growth. This desire has taken concrete, though perhaps temporary, form in the 1981 Budget Reconciliation Act, which reduces federal matching payments to states. More recently Congress has been considering various ways of reducing federal matching grants for specified types of services and beneficiaries. Other plans considered by the Reagan administration and the National Governors' Association have included proposals to federalize large portions of Medicaid and turn the remainder over to the states to be funded through block grants. Although such changes may produce some short-term budget savings or shifts, they do not get to the heart of Medicaid's problems and, as our evidence below suggests, may actually aggravate those problems. There has been little attempt by either Congress or the administration to specify how Medicaid costs can be cut (or their rate of increase slowed) in a way that is most consistent with the program's goals and does as little harm as possible to its beneficiaries.

In this study we analyze alternative long-term strategies for controlling Medicaid costs. We generally accept the premise, given projected deficits and the apparent consensus about national defense requirements, that the rate of growth in spending for social programs, including Medicaid, will have to be reduced. But our basic theme is equally applicable to tight and not-so-tight budget environments. In essence we are attempting to show how taxpayers can get the most for their Medicaid dollars, whatever the size of the Medicaid budget.

We take up two kinds of questions. In the first set are *positive* questions about the response of the system to policy parameters. We discuss what economic theory and empirical evidence have to say about probable outcomes under various policy alternatives. How would states respond to block grants? to a cap on federal Medicaid expenditures? to a reduction in the federal matching rate? What would be the implications of federalizing Medicaid? What are the likely effects of the various proposals for competition in the system, and how well would they work if applied to Medicaid? We pay particular attention to the effect such changes in federal policy would have on total expenditures, standards of eligibility, coverage, and the use of medical services by the poor.

Another set of questions addresses *normative* issues requiring value judgments. What should we be trying to accomplish with Medicaid? Who should receive Medicaid benefits? Who should pay for the program? We consider several alternative statements of what the social objectives ought to be and use them to define specific goals for Medicaid. Then we evaluate the various policy alternatives by their ability to achieve those goals. Our objective is to match program characteristics with social goals.

The major messages that emerge are simple. Cutting Medicaid outlays will necessarily reduce the well-being of beneficiaries to some extent; it is of no use to pretend that much saving can be wrung out of waste alone. But that effect on beneficiaries can be cushioned by changing the institutional arrangements of the program. In particular, a devolution of authority and control to state and local governments, providers, private sector insurers, and beneficiaries can help ensure that cuts are made where they do the least harm. Neither a fully federalized program nor an entirely state run program is likely to produce the best results, however. The proper balance will require continued, though modified, federal financial support and greater state responsibility for administration.

The successful implementation of this approach will call for two essential elements. First, states must be given the authority to make the kind of competition-oriented changes in their programs that will permit elimination of services of low marginal value to recipients. Limited ability to influence the use of services has been a major barrier to Medicaid cost control; and market-oriented innovations, such as vouchers and copayments, as well as conventional health maintenance organizations, provide the means for physicians and Medicaid beneficiaries themselves to make the choices about which services to do without.

The second requirement is that states be given financial incentives, embodied in matching rates or grants, to set Medicaid expenditures at levels consistent with both state and national preferences. Expenditures in each state should reflect national concern for equitable treatment of the poor in all states, and states that desire benefits much higher than the national average should provide them largely at their own expense. Thus competitive reforms would give states the *means* to reduce costs, and federal financial incentives would provide the *reason* for them to do so. Overall, this approach to Medicaid reform should result in a leaner, more equitable program with incentives for states, providers, and recipients to make better use of Medicaid resources.

4

2
Background of the Medicaid Problem

History of the Program

Why was the Medicaid program enacted? What objectives did Congress have in mind? These questions are controversial, in part because of the failure to separate rhetoric from fact. The generally accepted political explanation, ever since Medicaid was passed, has been that Medicaid was a kind of afterthought to Medicare. The American Medical Association had favored, in preference to Medicare, an extension of the Kerr-Mills program for the aged. After passage of the Medicare law was assured, the Kerr-Mills concept of joint federal-state financing was extended to the non-aged poor, partly, one suspects, to sop up the state funds that would otherwise have been released when the federal government assumed the financial burden for the aged under Medicare. Very little in the way of cost estimates, or even serious consideration of the implications of Medicaid, was done before its passage. The most one can say is that some vague sense of the desirability of broadening public programs for medical care for the poor and of making those programs more uniform and less dependent on state resources was responsible for the political decision.

Medicaid and Medicare both became effective in mid-1966. Although Medicare was fully federally financed and managed, Medicaid continued the pattern of federal-state financing of medical care for the poor of the Kerr-Mills program. As in that program, the federal share was inversely related to state per capita income. Kerr-Mills had continued a federal-state arrangement that had begun in 1950.

The major difference between Kerr-Mills and Medicaid was an extension of mandatory eligibility and federal sharing to welfare recipients who were not aged—that is, to recipients of Aid to Families with Dependent Children (AFDC)—who had previously been primarily a responsibility of the states alone. In addition, Medicaid provided an option for federal matching funds for care of the "medically needy" who were not eligible for welfare. Indeed, an original objective of Medicaid, later dropped, was to induce states to extend eligibility to all persons with income below a certain amount, regardless of whether their incomes were sufficiently low or their characteristics sufficiently special to qualify them for welfare.

Medicaid generally followed Medicare in basing reimbursement of providers on market prices or costs. State Medicaid programs were required to pay hospitals according to the Medicare cost-based standard, but they were permitted to pay physicians less than Medicare rates. Mandatory covered services, which could not be subject to copayment or deductible, were hospital care, physicians' services, diagnostic services, family planning consultation, and nursing home care in skilled nursing facilities. Screening and treatment of children were subsequently added. Optional items of coverage included care in intermediate-care facilities, dental care, drugs, eyeglasses, and some other medical services. Copayments were eventually permitted for some of these optional services and for hospital and physicians' services for the medically indigent.[1]

Mandatory eligibility is now required for persons receiving cash assistance under federally funded transfer programs. Therefore persons eligible for income transfers under AFDC are automatically eligible for Medicaid. States have considerable freedom in setting the income or other conditions for AFDC eligibility, however, and so can indirectly control the number eligible for Medicaid. Persons who are mandatory recipients of Supplemental Security Income (SSI), a federal program for the aged, blind, or disabled, are also automatically eligible for Medicaid. The income limits for SSI are set by the federal government.

Optional beneficiaries, for whom states may receive federal matching but whose coverage is not required by federal law, are those who are categorically eligible except that they do not receive, and may not be eligible for, cash assistance. This group includes medically needy families with dependent children whose incomes are above the state AFDC limit, as well as elderly persons not qualifying for cash assistance, many with large medical or nursing home bills.

The largest group of Medicaid recipients consists of dependent children under the age of twenty-one. But, as shown in table 2, this is also the group that is least costly (per recipient) to serve. Dependent children and the adults in their families constitute 65 percent of Medicaid recipients but are responsible for only about 28 percent of Medicaid expenditures. The largest share of Medicaid payments—37.5 percent—goes for services to the elderly, reflecting the cost of

TABLE 2

Medicaid Recipients and Payments by Eligibility Category, Fiscal Year 1980

Basis of Eligibility	Recipients		Payments[a]		Average Payment per Recipient (dollars)
	Number (thousands)	Percentage of total	Dollars (millions)	Percentage of total	
Age 65 or over	3,420	15.8	8,730	37.5	2,553
Blindness	92	0.4	131	0.6	1,424
Permanent and total disability	2,727	12.6	7,004	30.1	2,568
Dependent children under twenty-one	9,283	42.9	3,148	13.5	339
Adults in families with dependent children	4,784	22.1	3,357	14.4	702
Other	1,507	7.0	912	3.9	605
Total	21,617[b]	100.0[b]	23,283[c]	100.0	1,077

a. Payments are Medicaid vendor payments made to providers of service for care rendered to eligible individuals. Amounts include both state and federal share.

b. Categories do not add to totals because of a small number of recipients who are in more than one category during the year.

c. Detail does not add to total because of rounding.

Source: "HCFA Program Statistics," *Health Care Financing Review*, vol. 3, no. 3 (March 1982), pp. 123-24.

long-term nursing home services as well as the greater need for medical services of this group. The disabled category, which includes terminally ill persons under age sixty-five and mentally retarded persons as well as low-income persons with work-related disabilities, includes less than 13 percent of recipients but accounts for about 30 percent of Medicaid payments.

The most commonly used Medicaid services are—as shown in table 3—prescribed drugs and physicians' services. Hospital out-patient services are used by more than 44 percent of recipients, particularly those in inner-city areas with access to the typically large ambulatory care units of teaching hospitals. The proportion of primary care provided by physicians in private practice is much lower for Medicaid recipients than for the population as a whole. Inpatient hospital services are used by about 17 percent of Medicaid recipients each year.

TABLE 3

Medicaid Recipients and Payments by Type of Service, Fiscal Year 1980

Service	Recipients Using Service		Payments		Average Payment per Recipient (dollars)
	Number (thousands)	Percentage of total	Dollars (millions)	Percentage of total	
Inpatient hospitals	3,742	17.3	6,261	26.9	1,673
Mental hospitals	67	0.3	873	3.7	13,030
Nursing homes (SNFs and nonmental ICFs)[a]	1,399	6.5	7,930	34.1	5,668
ICF—mentally retarded	125	0.6	1,975	8.5	15,800
Physicians' services	13,795	63.8	1,869	8.0	135
Dental services	4,638	21.5	462	2.0	99
Other practitioners' services	3,173	14.7	195	0.8	61
Outpatient hospital services	9,583	44.3	1,101	4.7	115
Clinic services	1,571	7.3	321	1.4	204
Laboratory and radiological services	3,399	15.7	121	0.5	36
Home health services	393	1.8	332	1.4	845
Prescribed drugs	13,810	63.9	1,321	5.7	96
Family planning services	1,120	5.2	82	0.4	73
Other care	2,447	11.3	441	1.9	180
All services	21,617[b]		23,283	100.0	1,077

a. SNF = skilled nursing facility; ICF = intermediate-care facility.
b. Detail does not add to total because of recipients who use more than one service.
Source: "HCFA Program Statistics" (March 1982).

Among services the largest share of Medicaid payments (73 percent) goes for care in institutions, including hospitals, mental hospitals, nursing homes, and intermediate-care facilities for the mentally retarded (ICFs-MR). Medicaid payments per user are largest in mental hospitals and ICFs-MR because stays in such institutions are frequently long. Medicaid payments per user of nursing home services are somewhat lower, since elderly recipients usually have some income and are required to contribute nearly all of it to the cost of care before Medicaid will pay.

TABLE 4

Payments for Medical Care, by Source, 1980, and Rate of Growth, 1977–1980

Source of Payment	1980 Payments ($ billions)	Annual Rate of Growth 1977–1980[a]
Private health insurance	64.6	17.4
Medicare[b]	33.3	16.7
Medicaid[c]	23.3	12.7

a. Annual compound rate of growth as a percentage.

b. Bills approved for payment. Figures may slightly understate rate of growth to the extent that some 1980 bills may not have been approved by the cutoff date for these data (fall 1981).

c. Medicaid vendor payments.

SOURCES: Computed from "HCFA Program Statistics," *Health Care Financing Review*, vol. 4, no. 1 (September 1982); and *Source Book of Health Insurance Data 1981-1982*.

The alacrity with which some states initially accepted Medicaid was exceeded only by their generosity with part-federal dollars in the program's early years, especially in such high-income states as New York and California. Then began a gradual but accelerating race to see whether federal and state attempts to control costs could offset the increase in recipients as more and more people tried to sign up.

In recent years state efforts have, in fact, been effective in keeping the rate of growth in Medicaid expenditures below that of private health insurance and the federally administered Medicare program (see table 4). In part this is because states have been successful in curbing the growth in the number of recipients by choosing not to adjust income eligibility standards upward fully to keep pace with inflation. As shown in table 5, recent growth in Medicaid costs has been due to general inflation, the more rapid price increases in the medical care sector (partially resulting from greater service intensity), and increases in the quantity of services used per recipient. The results reflect the existing program structure under which states have had little ability to influence prices paid for services (except physicians' services) or to limit use by recipients. Cost-based reimbursement has been the rule for hospitals, and, even where prospective rates have been used (most frequently for nursing homes), this year's costs generally determine next year's rates. States have not

9

TABLE 5

SOURCES OF GROWTH IN MEDICAID COSTS, 1977–1980

	Annual Rate of Growth[a] (percent)	Relative Contribution to Cost Increase (percent)
General inflation[b]	8.3	66
Extra inflation in medical care prices[c]	1.3	10
Number of recipients	−1.9	−16
Use per recipient[d]	4.9	39
Total[e]	12.7	100

a. Annual compound rate of growth 1977-1980.

b. Based on GNP deflator.

c. Based on medical care component of the consumer price index minus GNP deflator.

d. Includes effect of shift toward a greater proportion of recipients in the disabled category.

e. Detail does not add to total because of rounding and second-order effects of growth.

SOURCES: Computed by authors using data from *Statistical Abstract of the United States 1981* and "HCFA Program Statistics" (March 1982).

been allowed to require copayments by most recipients for the major services, and, although Medicaid recipients may be given the option of using a health maintenance organization, states have not been able to give them an incentive to do so when care is available elsewhere at no out-of-pocket cost. The one thing states have been able to control effectively is eligibility, and this is reflected in the recent decline in the number of recipients. It may even be that cost-conscious states have been forced to squeeze harder in this area than they would like; if effective means were found to reduce use and cost per recipient, states might be willing to expand eligibility to some extent.

Most of the recent increases in Medicaid payments have gone to the aged and the disabled. As shown in table 6, in the period 1977–1980, 36 percent of the total growth in Medicaid payments was for disabled persons, and 41 percent was for other persons over age sixty-five. The blind and the disabled are the only categories of persons eligible for Medicaid in which the number of recipients has been growing. The growth in the disabled category may reflect a number of influences. There is evidence that increases

TABLE 6

GROWTH IN MEDICAID PAYMENTS, RECIPIENTS, AND SERVICES AND
SHARES OF TOTAL COST INCREASE, BY BASIS OF ELIGIBILITY,
FISCAL YEARS 1977–1980

	Rate of Growth (percent)[a]				Percentage of Total Medicaid Cost Increase
Basis of Eligibility	Payments	Number of recipients	Payments per recipient	Service per recipient[b]	
Age 65 or over	14.4	−1.8	16.5	6.4	41.4
Blindness	6.3	0.4	5.9	−3.3	0.3
Disability	16.3	0.5	15.7	5.6	36.4
Children under 21	8.7	−1.5	10.4	0.8	10.0
Adults in families with dependent children	9.9	−0.1	10.0	0.4	11.8
Other	0.1	−9.5	10.7	1.0	0.0 +
All recipients	12.7	−1.9	14.9	4.9	100.0[c]

a. Annual compound rate of growth 1977-1980.

b. Computed from payments per recipient adjusted for growth in the medical care component of the consumer price index.

c. Detail does not add to total because of rounding.

SOURCE: Computed by authors from data in "HCFA Program Statistics" (March 1982).

in social security disability payments have led some persons—particularly those with low income potential—to leave the labor market, and some of these show up on Medicaid rolls.[2] But overall the growth in the number of persons receiving disability compensation has moderated.[3] A more significant source of growth in Medicaid payments for the disabled is the recent trend toward deinstitutionalization of the mentally retarded. As shown in table 7, the rate of growth in Medicaid recipients using intermediate-care facilities (ICFs) for the mentally retarded has been greater than that for any other service. When the mentally retarded leave state institutions, they may become eligible for Medicaid benefits in ICFs or in the community. The resulting increase in Medicaid expenditures comes from shifting costs from state-funded institutions to the federal-state Medicaid program and in many cases from an upgrading from the largely custodial care of state institutions to the more "habilitative" type of care in Medicaid-funded ICFs.

TABLE 7

GROWTH IN MEDICAID PAYMENTS AND RECIPIENTS AND SHARES OF TOTAL
COST INCREASE, BY TYPE OF SERVICE, FISCAL YEARS 1977–1980
(percent)

	Rate of Growth[a]			Share of Total Medicaid Cost Increase
	Payments	Number of recipients	Payments per recipient	
Inpatient hospitals	10.8	−0.3	11.2	23.7
Mental hospitals	14.7	−7.3	23.7	4.2
Nursing homes (SNFs and nonmental ICFs)[b]	14.1	0.5	13.6	37.0
ICF—mentally retarded	31.4	7.4	22.4	15.8
Physicians' services	7.0	−5.1	12.7	4.9
Dental services	2.5	0.0	2.5	0.5
Other practitioners' services	7.3	2.5	4.7	0.5
Outpatient hospital services	7.6	3.4	4.0	3.1
Clinic services	23.4	−1.9	25.8	2.1
Laboratory and radiological services	11.9	−14.9	3.5	−0.8
Home health services	22.6	2.0	20.2	2.2
Prescribed drugs	8.7	−3.6	12.8	4.2
Family planning services	−11.4	−5.9	−5.9	−0.5
Other care	26.7	−9.2	39.5	3.2
All services	12.7	−1.9	14.9	100.0[c]

a. Annual compound rate of growth 1977-1980.
b. SNF = skilled nursing facility; ICF = intermediate-care facility.
c. Detail does not add to total because of rounding.
SOURCE: Computed from data in "HCFA Program Statistics" (March 1982).

Although the aging of the nation's population has received much attention in the press, it has yet to show up as a dominating force in increasing Medicaid expenditures. The number of recipients over age sixty-five actually declined in the period 1977–1980. The growing number of elderly persons is a problem that will have to be faced in the future. Increasing use of services by elderly recipients, however, has been responsible for about 41 percent of recent growth in Medicaid costs. Care for the elderly in ICFs is a rapidly growing component of Medicaid (16.8 percent per year in this period), but costs for skilled nursing facilities (SNFs) have been growing somewhat more slowly than the average rate for Medicaid. This may reflect some substitution of a lower level of care for cases that might otherwise have been cared for in an SNF. Nevertheless, as shown in table 7, when SNFs, and ICFs are considered together, the rate of growth of nursing home costs has been somewhat greater than the rate for Medicaid costs as a whole.

Over 80 percent of the increase in Medicaid costs during the period 1977–1980 can be attributed to institutional care, including services of acute care and mental hospitals, SNFs, and mental and other ICFs. Increases in payments to nursing homes alone account for 37 percent of the growth in Medicaid payments during the period. Although growth in the number of Medicaid recipients using nursing homes accounts for a small portion of this increase, most of it has resulted from an increase in payments per recipient, which in turn reflects a rise in the average reimbursement rate for a day of nursing home care. Since the Omnibus Reconciliation Act of 1980, states have been able to reimburse nursing homes at "reasonable and adequate" rates rather than the "reasonable cost-related" rates previously used. The change was intended to give state Medicaid agencies somewhat more flexibility in setting rates. It is not yet clear whether this moderate relaxation of federal requirements will have much impact on Medicaid payments for nursing home services.

Changes in Medicaid patients' patterns of using hospital services are evident in table 8. The average length of stay has declined dramatically, but this decline has been offset by an increase in the frequency of hospitalizations (discharges) that greatly exceeds the increase in discharges per capita in the United States. Physicians may have responded to pressure from professional standards review organizations (PSROs) to get their patients out of the hospital sooner, but Medicaid provides no incentive for physicians or their patients to seek alternatives to hospital admission.

Payments for clinic services and home health services have been growing rapidly. They constitute only a small portion of total Medicaid payments, however, and hence account for only a small share of the recent growth in Medicaid expenditures. The rate of growth in payments for physicians' services, which have not involved cost-based reimbursement, has been much less than the rates for other components. State limits on reimbursement and the resulting decrease in the number of recipients using physicians' services (as physicians refuse to serve Medicaid patients) are contributing factors. Similarly payments for (and use of) hospital outpatient services, which had previously grown rapidly, have recently been increasing more slowly, perhaps partly in response to more restrictive reimbursement policies in some states.

TABLE 8

Medicaid Payments for Hospital Services and Related Factors, 1975 and 1979

	1975	1979	Annual Rate of Growth 1975–1979[a]
Payments ($ thousands)	3,411	5,650	13.4
CPI hospital component	236.1	370.3	11.9
Number of users (thousands)	3,436	3,742	2.2
Discharges (thousands)	4,508	6,060	7.7
Discharges per hospital user[b]	1.31	1.62	5.4
Discharges per Medicaid recipient	0.205	0.285	8.6
Days of care (thousands)	34,122	35,343	0.9
Average length of stay (days)	7.57	5.83	−6.3
Payment per day (dollars)	99.96	159.86	12.5
Payment per stay (dollars)	756.65	932.34	5.4

a. Annual compound percentage rate of growth.
b. Medicaid recipients using hospital services.
Sources: Donald Muse and Darwin Sawyer, *The Medicare and Medicaid Data Book, 1981*, HCFA, April 1982; *Statistical Abstract of the United States 1981*; and "HCFA Program Statistics," *Health Care Financing Review*, vol. 3, no. 4 (June 1982).

There is an important message here for controlling costs. Cutting Medicaid costs requires tackling the faults the program shares with the general health insurance system and will probably necessitate making Medicaid reimbursement mechanisms different from those of conventional insurance. Since recent growth in Medicaid costs has come mainly from inflation in medical care prices and increased use per recipient, these are the most likely areas for cost-saving measures. Reducing the growth in prices paid for services will require unlinking Medicaid from the system of cost reimbursement by third-party payers that has helped drive prices in the U.S. medical care system up faster than general inflation. Second, means must be found to limit use by recipients. There is little evidence that Medicaid recipients have used services more than other persons with full insurance coverage, nor is there evidence of greater "fat" or "waste" in provision of services under Medicaid than under other public or private programs. Cuts in Medicaid, therefore, will not be completely painless; they will mean giving up some services.

Effect on Use and Health

The stated goal of Medicaid, as an in-kind transfer program, has been to "provide medical assistance to [those] whose income and resources are insufficient to meet the cost of necessary medical services." The program has been successful in increasing consumption of medical care by the eligible poor. It has been associated with growth in the use of visits to physicians, hospital admissions, and hospital days by beneficiaries and therefore by poor people generally.

Since the initiation of Medicaid, there has been a shift in patterns of use, so that low-income persons now visit physicians more often than those with higher incomes. A smaller fraction of those visits, however, are to physicians in private offices and relatively more are to hospital outpatient departments. Among the poor population, visit rates tend to be higher for those receiving Medicaid, but Medicaid recipients tend to be sicker than the poor in general. An adjustment for health status in 1969 data by Davis and Reynolds suggests that the poor receiving public assistance, including Medicaid, use physicians' services slightly more frequently than other persons. But the poor without aid see physicians at a much lower rate—so much so that the health-status-adjusted rates are lower for the poor in general, especially for children and the elderly.[4] No more recent adjusted data are available, but there is no reason to think that the situation has changed much since 1969.

In short, Medicaid has reduced inequality in the use of physicians' services and has contributed to greater use of hospital care by the poor. But there still remain differences in use—for the poor who are not on Medicaid, and related to race and location—so we cannot say that access is equal. Indeed, much of the remaining inequality is an indirect product of Medicaid, reflecting interstate variations in Medicaid eligibility requirements and benefits.

But has Medicaid increased the use of "necessary" medical services? If necessary medical services are defined as those that improve health, matters are not so clear. The effect of Medicaid on health is hard to determine, much less to quantify. Some facts are not in dispute. There have been fairly pronounced improvements in many indicators of the nation's health since 1965, the year Medicaid legislation was passed—but the improvements are largely a continuation of pre-1965 trends. Death rates from heart diseases, diabetes, and most other causes except lung cancer have declined, as they have been declining since 1945. But much of the evidence we have suggests that mortality is more directly related to income, education, and life style than to additional medical care.[5] Since the research

15

results so far available are not based on randomized experiments, we cannot be sure that self-selection in the use of medical services does not lead to an understatement of the effect of those services. The lack of a positive correlation between medical care and health may occur because causality moves in two opposing directions—poor health resulting in greater use of medical care and medical care improving health. That is, the effect of medical services on health may be obscured by the fact that persons with poor health need to use more medical services.

Jack Hadley has attempted to deal with this problem using a production-of-health model. He concludes that "greater medical care use is a significant factor in explaining lower mortality rates."[6] Because only limited data on medical care use are available for the county groups of Hadley's analysis, he employs average Medicare expenditures per person enrolled as a proxy measure of use and relies on the assumption that this measure is proportional to actual use for each age-race-sex cohort investigated. Medicare expenditures may be a good proxy for Medicare-covered services used by the elderly, but it is less clear what Hadley's results may mean for nonelderly age groups or for the services such as long-term nursing home care that Medicaid pays for on behalf of elderly recipients. Gerontologists have suggested that nursing home placement, rather than improving health, often contributes to poor psychological well-being and reduced functional capacity. For those elderly Medicaid recipients with nearby relatives, much of the benefit of Medicaid-covered nursing home care may accrue to relatives who would have provided care at home or paid for services themselves. While financial relief for such families (poor and nonpoor) may be desirable, we would not expect to find major positive effects on health for this portion of Medicaid expenditures. Because Medicaid coverage is different from that of Medicare, its health effects may differ as well.

Because no aggregate data are yet available on death rates by income class, attempts to examine effects on the poor people Medicaid assists must use proxy measures for poverty in addition to imperfect measures of health. One such imperfect proxy is race, since a higher proportion of nonwhites are poor. (This proxy must be used with caution because there may be special racial effects as well.) A comparison of mortality rates by race and sex for the period 1965–1977 shows no persistent pattern of differences by race. Nor do we have other evidence that Medicaid, or even the use of medical care generally, has had a major effect on mortality rates for poor adults.

For infants, children, and mothers—special targets of Medicaid and the war-on-poverty programs that accompanied it—there is a bit more evidence. The rates of fetal deaths, neonatal deaths, infant deaths, and maternal deaths all declined by larger percentages in the period 1965–1970 than in the preceding five years. And in all four cases, the decline was larger in absolute value and in percentage for blacks than for whites. Thus, at least for infants, there is evidence that something happened about 1965. The Medicaid program was almost certainly a contributing factor, but other causes may have been more important. The decline in infant mortality might be linked to the sharp drop in fertility rates that took place in the late 1960s, particularly for women over age thirty-five. Another possible explanation lies in changes in the economic well-being of the poor, particularly of poor blacks, brought about by social changes in the 1960s and the Great Society programs of which Medicaid was only a part.

In a study of variations in infant mortality rates among U.S. counties, Michael Grossman and Steven Jacobowitz found the increase in the legal abortion rate and increased use of organized family planning by low-income women to be the most important factors explaining reductions in nonwhite neonatal mortality rates in the period 1964–1971. They also found weaker evidence that maternal and infant care projects—state-administered programs with federal and state funding but not part of Medicaid—contributed slightly to the decline in neonatal mortality rates.[7] This is consistent with earlier evidence of low mortality rates for children of poor women in maternal and infant projects relative to supposedly comparable groups.[8]

Other changes in medicine or the delivery of medical care might also be responsible for the striking improvements in the survival rates of low-birth-weight infants.[9] For the period immediately after birth, the hospital and what it does appear to be the primary determinants of mortality rates. Hospital neonatal care units can now save a significant fraction of premature infants even under two pounds— though sometimes with lasting birth defects. It may well be, therefore, that technical progress in the care of newborns is responsible for much of the decline in neonatal mortality rates. Yet hospitalization for delivery was generally available to the poor even before Medicaid; so this care probably would have been provided anyway. Nevertheless, Medicaid has played a role in paying for intensive neonatal care, with costs that can range from $20,000 to $200,000 for very low weight infants.

Recently there have been upturns in the infant mortality rate in some localities hard hit by the recession, but these appear to be more closely related to falling income than to loss of Medicaid benefits. For example, press reports have attributed hospitalization and some infant deaths to substitution of regular milk or even sugar water for baby formula by low-income mothers trying to save money. Here the best solution would seem to be greater emphasis on income maintenance, health education, and nutrition rather than medical care. The postnatal parts of programs such as Title V maternal and child health block grants and WIC, a program that provides infant formula and diet supplements to poor women, may be better suited than Medicaid for these purposes and may even help save Medicaid costs.

Direct evidence of Medicaid's effect on the health of recipients is limited and conflicting. Friedman, Parker, and Lipworth found no effect of either Medicaid or private health insurance on early diagnosis of breast cancer.[10] Kehrer and Wolin found no significant effect of Medicaid eligibility on birth weight of infants born to participants in the Gary income maintenance experiment.[11] Grossman and Jacobowitz provide evidence that Medicaid coverage of first pregnancies accounts for about 7 percent of the reduction in neonatal mortality rates for nonwhites between 1964 and 1977, but their evidence suggests that such coverage is associated with higher neonatal mortality rates for whites.[12] The conflicting results of these studies are not surprising given that available data do not permit researchers to control, either experimentally or econometrically, for the many and varied individual and environmental factors that affect health outcomes.

In summary, there are few improvements reflected in conventional health statistics that can be clearly attributed to Medicaid; but it should be recognized that this is not the same as saying that Medicaid has had no effect on health. We assume the program has beneficial effects even if they are difficult to measure. What does all of this suggest about places to cut Medicaid costs and do the least damage to health? General health effects seem most likely to be found in infants, and for them hospital care may be more important than other services. For older children and adults, some cuts could probably be made in Medicaid expenditures without discernible effects on health indicators. But it should be emphasized that this does *not* mean that cuts will not make some people worse off or will not affect health at all.

The main conclusion is that there are no strong indicators about which, if any, components of the Medicaid program significantly affect the health of the poor. Nor do the professional experts really know which cuts in Medicaid benefits would have the smallest adverse effects. At the moment, therefore, there is no basis for trying to direct states to trim their Medicaid programs in any particular way. With the prevailing uncertainty about what is best, giving states the flexibility to experiment and adapt their cost controlling efforts to local circumstances, and to develop incentives for physicians and patients to control costs, may be the most sensible policy.

Notes

1. For more background on the Medicaid program in its early years, see Robert Stevens and Rosemary Stevens, *Welfare Medicine in America: A Case Study of Medicaid* (New York: Free Press, 1974).

2. See Donald O. Parsons, "The Decline in Male Labor Force Participation," *Journal of Political Economy*, vol. 88, no. 1 (February 1980), pp. 117–34; and Howard P. Marvel, "An Economic Analysis of the Operation of Social Security Disability Insurance," *Journal of Human Resources*, vol. 18, no. 3 (Summer 1982), pp. 393–412.

3. Congressional Budget Office, "Disability Compensation: Current Issues and Options for Changes," June 1982.

4. Karen Davis and Roger Reynolds, "The Impact of Medicare and Medicaid on Access to Medical Care," in Richard N. Rosett, ed., *The Role of Health Insurance in the Health Services Sector* (New York: National Bureau of Economic Research, 1976).

5. See Victor R. Fuchs, *Who Shall Live? Health, Economics, and Social Choice* (New York: Basic Books, 1974), chaps. 1, 2; Joseph P. Newhouse and Lindy J. Friedlander, "The Relationship between Medical Resources and Measures of Health," *Journal of Human Resources*, vol. 15, no. 2 (Spring 1980), pp. 200–218; Lee Benham and Alexandra Benham, "The Impact of Incremental Medical Services on Health Status 1963–1970," in Ronald Anderson et al., *Equity in Health Services: Empirical Analysis in Social Policy* (Cambridge, Mass.: Ballinger, 1975).

6. Jack Hadley, *More Medical Care, Better Health?: An Economic Analysis of Mortality Rates* (Washington, D.C.: Urban Institute, 1982).

7. Michael Grossman and Steven Jacobowitz, "Variations in Infant Mortality Rates among Counties of the United States: The Roles of Public Policies and Programs," *Demography*, vol. 18, no. 4 (November 1981).

8. See Karen Davis and Kathy Schoen, *Health and the War on Poverty* (Washington, D.C.: Brookings Institution, 1978). These comparisons do not take into account possible self-selection of more conscientious or healthier mothers into the programs.

9. Jeffrey Harris, "Prenatal Care and Infant Mortality," in Victor Fuchs, ed., *Economic Aspects of Health* (Chicago: University of Chicago Press, 1982), pp. 15–51, contrasts this with comparatively little change in the proportion of low-birth-weight infants and relatively weak evidence of the effectiveness of prenatal care on birth weight.

10. Bernard Friedman, Paul Parker, and Leslie Lipworth, "The Influence of Medicaid and Private Health Insurance on the Early Diagnosis of Breast Cancer," *Medical Care*, vol. 1 (November–December 1973), pp. 485–90.

11. Barbara Kehrer and Charles Wolin, "Impact of Income Maintenance on Low Birth Weight: Evidence from the Gary Experiment," *Journal of Human Resources*, vol. 14, no. 4 (Fall 1979).

12. Michael Grossman and Steven Jacobowitz, "Variations in Infant Mortality Rates." Coverage of first-time pregnancies was the only aspect of the Medicaid program investigated in this study, and the effects found for Medicaid are not highly significant statistically. Confirmation of this effect and the abortion law effect reported above is provided by Hadley, *More Medical Care, Better Health?*

3
Problems of the Current Medicaid Program

Has Medicaid been a success or a failure? What are the problems of the program as it stands? The failure of the political process to make Medicaid's goals clear obviously contributes to imprecise evaluation, but an analysis of the desirability of changes can best proceed only after we have identified the problems that need correcting. In this chapter we discuss some outcomes of the program that have been considered problems. We attempt to sort out those that are fundamental and need direct treatment from those that are only symptomatic of the more basic problems and can be expected to disappear if other needed changes are made in the program's design.

Exclusion of Some Low-Income Persons from Eligibility

Because eligibility for Medicaid is based on being aged, blind, disabled, or in a family receiving benefits from Aid to Families with Dependent Children, there are numerous persons in households with incomes below the poverty line who are not eligible for Medicaid.[1] The ineligible poor tend to be able-bodied individuals between ages twenty-one and sixty-four, childless couples, or two-parent families. Because many states have income limits for AFDC that are below the U.S. poverty level, many poor people fit the categories but are still not eligible. We limit our discussion in this section, however, to those excluded because they do not fit in the eligible categories.

Many of us would regard the categorical exclusion of some poor families as a problem, but why? Another way of asking the same question is to ask why Congress has so far limited Medicaid eligibility to persons in particular categories. The answer, one suspects, is that there is a desire to limit aid to the *deserving* poor, that is, to those who are poor through no fault of their own. Part of the reason for this limitation is undoubtedly moralistic: indolence ought not to be rewarded. But part of it may have to do with economic efficiency. Work effort is unlikely to be affected by transfers to those whose poverty is purely involuntary. For households with both parents present or for non-aged, nondisabled single individuals, however, low income could be the result of voluntary choices about work effort or, at worst, temporary misfortune. In such cases, it is feared that work effort and economic output would fall if poverty were rewarded with transfers either of income, as with AFDC, or of goods and services in kind, as with Medicaid. Then do Medicaid's categorical eligibility requirements make sense?

Ultimately, part of the answer to this question is empirical—concerning how much of the poverty of various categories of the poor is voluntary, a reflection of employment choices. Part also depends on the preferences of donor-taxpayers—how much poverty are they willing to pay to alleviate, at what cost? After all, for a person who could not work in any case, a dollar transferred results in a dollar of added income, but a dollar transferred to someone who is capable of working and who therefore reduces his work effort leads to less than a dollar of added income. Taxpayers may be willing to pay a dollar to increase recipients' benefits by a dollar but not to increase net benefits (after work response) by something less than a dollar.

The question of categorical eligibility for Medicaid is therefore related to the larger question of appropriate income transfers and their effect on work effort. There is, however, one difference. For income transfers, there seems no particular reason why the "ideal" income should depend on the categories for eligibility; that is, a family eligible for AFDC seems to have no greater need for total income than an otherwise similar family that is not eligible. One can reasonably argue, however, that the socially desirable amount of medical insurance support is greater for households with a greater need for medical services. Consequently, the eligibility for an ideal public program ought to take into account more than just income in relation to the poverty line. In particular, it surely ought to take into account the needs of the disabled and the elderly. The present Medicaid eligibility categories reflect our efforts to concentrate benefits on groups with the greatest need and the least work response. Perhaps, despite their faults, the categories do make some sense, although we must recognize that they are a very crude and imperfect means of separating the deserving from the undeserving poor.

We can, however, say that the all-or-nothing nature of the Medicaid program seems hard to square with reality. It is simply not plausible that the categorically eligible do not reduce their work effort at all, while the ineligible would reduce their work effort so much as to justify no assistance. Indeed, comparatively large labor supply responses were found for female household heads in some

22

income maintenance experiments.[2] It is also possible to get into categories defined by household structure voluntarily. Despite greater availability of birth control, between 1965 and 1979 births to unmarried women increased from 26.3 to 48.8 percent of all births among nonwhites and more than doubled from 4.0 to 9.4 percent among whites. And between 1959 and 1979—a period in which the total number of persons below the poverty level declined by 36 percent—the number of poor in female-headed households with no husband present increased by 25 percent. While there have been many social and economic changes in the past two decades, one wonders what effect the categorical eligibility rules of the current welfare system, including Medicaid, may have had in encouraging the formation of one-parent families. Considering the incentives for all involved, a reasonable compromise might be to have less generous benefits and somewhat more restrictive income standards and work requirements for the currently ineligible poor (including single individuals and two-parent families) than for the categorically eligible but to provide them with some access to assistance, perhaps for catastrophic illnesses or perhaps in the form of a subsidized insurance plan. An alternative for those with a work history would be to require catastrophic health insurance, paid for during periods of working, that carried a sufficiently high premium to carry through periods of unemployment.

Variation in Eligibility Standards and Benefits

Interstate differences in Medicaid eligibility and benefits are sizable. A poor person with given income, assets, and family situation may be eligible for assistance if he lives in one state but not if he lives in another. In some states only a fraction of persons below the poverty level receive Medicaid; in other states large numbers of nonpoor receive benefits.[3] The Congressional Budget Office estimates that in 1980 about 16 million people with annual incomes above the federal poverty guidelines were eligible for Medicaid during some portion of the year.[4] To some extent the variation in income limits mirrors variation in the cost of living, so that real income limits vary less than nominal ones. But real income standards and other criteria for eligibility do nevertheless vary considerably; in fact, we estimate that real income standards vary by a factor of 5.[5] The unequal eligibility criteria imply that Medicaid is characterized by horizontal inequity (that is, treats similar people in similar circumstances unequally) and fails to allocate its resources to the most needy.

States also vary considerably in Medicaid benefits per recipient. Table C-2 in appendix C shows how payments per recipient vary among states for three categories of recipients. There is a direct relationship between state income and the amount of benefits.[6] This suggests that, although the current matching-rate formula is a function of income, it has not been properly adjusted to equalize benefits. There is evidence that some of the interstate differences in benefits may simply reflect the lower demand for Medicaid in states with lower taxpayer income. To a large degree it may be low income and other economic factors including inappropriate matching rates, rather than lack of generosity or different attitudes toward the poor, that have led to lower Medicaid benefits in many southern states.

Together the variations in eligibility standards and benefit levels imply correspondingly large disparities in the average benefit per poor person. In 1980 Medicaid payments per poor person ranged from $315 in Florida to $1,938 in New York. Adjusting for price differences, real benefits per poor person in New Mexico were only 16 percent of those in Wisconsin (see table C–1 in appendix C).

Why are the differences in benefits regarded as a problem? One reason is that there may be, in a sense to be discussed in more detail later, a concern by persons elsewhere in the country for the well-being of the poor in all states, including those with strict eligibility standards. We might all feel better if medical care were provided to the most needy first, regardless of their state of residence.

Another reason to favor more nearly equal benefits is that differences in eligibility and benefits set up incentives for people to move to those states with the most generous programs. These movements have real and explicit economic costs. Again using the imperfect proxy of race for income, we find that many states with high Medicaid and AFDC benefits—including Massachusetts, New York, Connecticut, Wisconsin, and California—experienced a high net rate of immigration of blacks in the 1960s, both in total and in relation to whites. In the same period many low-benefit states—including Mississippi, South Carolina, and New Mexico—experienced a large out-migration of blacks.[7] Although other factors also lie behind the aggregate numbers, interstate variation in welfare programs, including Medicaid, may be at least partly responsible.[8] If so, one adverse effect of the program has been to attract the poor to areas with relatively high costs of living, where in consequence the public or private cost of their maintenance is higher. Many high-benefit states also tend to have higher than average rates of unemployment, making the opportunities for getting off the welfare system more limited. A more nearly equal distribution of benefits, which would not produce such incentives for people to move, appears to be in the best interests of taxpayers and Medicaid beneficiaries alike.

Variations in the Tax Burden among States

While the tax burden of the federal portion of Medicaid costs is distributed according to the progressive federal tax structure, the distribution of the burden for taxpayers of the state share reflects the wide variation in state Medicaid programs and state resources. The share of a taxpayer's income that goes to Medicaid depends on the generosity of the state program, the number of poor people in the state, the number and wealth of other taxpayers in the state, state business and resource tax collections, and the state's tax structure, as well as the state's federal Medicaid matching rate. But the federal matching rate varies only with state per capita income and is not directly adjusted for state resources in relation to the needs of the poor. For this reason, many low-income states with high poverty rates and low tax bases have been forced to choose between an above-average tax burden and below-average benefits. In most cases they have chosen the latter. If Mississippi, for example, were to expand Medicaid benefits per poor person to the national average at current matching rates, the share of state taxpayers' income devoted to Medicaid would exceed the national average. Moreover, as we point out below, the income elasticity of state demand for Medicaid appears to be somewhat greater than unity. So we would expect states of relatively low income to prefer to spend a smaller share of taxpayers' income on the program. The current matching rates do not adequately compensate for these natural differences in states' responses. Thus, with current matching rates, the potential tax burden of expanded programs is a barrier to more nearly equal benefits among states.

The northeastern states, in contrast, have fared reasonably well under the current form of Medicaid. Although many states in the Northeast have relatively high incomes and hence lower federal matching rates, the lower matching rates have been more than offset by the higher benefits and greater expenditures to which matching applies. Federal Medicaid payments per capita are consequently much higher in the Northeast, and Medicaid has produced a net redistribution of resources to that region from other parts of the country.[9] The unequal tax burdens and distribution of federal funds create incentives for taxpayers to move to states where the burden of supporting the poor is relatively low. In some marginal cases this may mean turning down higher-paying jobs where they would be more productive. Thus for taxpayers as well as for recipients there are both equity and efficiency reasons for concern.

State Fiscal Distress

Some states have had fiscal difficulties that have been blamed on high or increasing Medicaid costs. It is difficult to determine whether this is a different problem from those already discussed or just a manifestation of them. Fiscal distress—the failure to match expenditures with taxes—can come about, of course, either because expenditures are too high or because taxes are too low.

Some states have apparently underestimated the cost of Medicaid. Because expenditures on entitlement programs such as Medicaid depend on economic conditions, they cannot be predicted precisely, but errors in forecasts should average out over time. There is no reason state policy makers should *consistently* underestimate future expenditures, except possibly for political purposes. State expenditures for other programs such as unemployment compensation are probably even less predictable than Medicaid and hence may be a more important cause of fiscal distress.

Other states having established a Medicaid program may find that they have difficulty in raising the taxes to pay for it, even when expenditures are forecasted correctly. Politicians may fear voters' disapproval of higher taxes. Or they may fear out-migration of taxpayers and businesses. But their own real alternatives are clear: to scuttle the Medicaid program or to grit their teeth and go ahead with higher taxes or fewer other services. One may wish that public services cost less, but wishing will not make it so. "Fiscal distress" is thus not a root cause but only a symptom of the other diseases we are discussing.

State fiscal distress is partly a product of the way federal-state programs are financed—how costs are divided between federal, state, and local payers. If states are judged to be spending too much relative to the federal government, financial arrangements can be altered easily enough. The solution need not involve federalization of program administrative functions. It should be kept in mind, however, that using federal borrowing or local property taxes to substitute for state dollars is like substituting one tax for another. All of this discussion depends crucially on the interpretation of macroeconomic considerations: a budgetary deficit is not, in itself, a reason to avoid financing an additional expenditure for desired services, however politically distasteful further deficits or tax increases may be. In this study we avoid dealing directly with the problems of matching state expenditures with revenues. What we consider, however, is how various options for federal-state financing of Medicaid would affect state tax burdens. We believe the issue of whether state or federal spending is too high or too low is best resolved by the political process, and we leave it to others.

High and Growing Program Costs

The cost of Medicaid is probably the most fundamental issue, a problem in itself and an exacerbating influence on all the other problems. There are two aspects of the problem, which need to be distinguished throughout our analysis. Costs are high and rising, some say, because of "fat" in the system—pure inefficiency, an inability to get the maximum real benefits out of the tax dollars being spent. Their hope is that if somehow this fat could be excised, we could cut cost without lowering quality or access, or we could improve benefits, or we could expand eligibility, or we could do a little bit of all three. As already mentioned, we take a pessimistic view of the potential for reducing this kind of inefficiency.

The second possibility is that high and rising costs per recipient do indeed reflect higher real benefits—in quantity or quality—but benefits for which taxpayers are unwilling to pay the price. To a considerable extent improvements in quality, largely fed by the third-party reimbursement system, have proceeded at about the same pace in Medicaid as in the medical care sector generally. It would be difficult to redirect the growth of medical care technology with Medicaid program changes alone from the current cost-increasing, quality-enhancing variety toward the cost-reducing kind, although this might be possible with systemwide competitive reforms. So unless we are willing to deny Medicaid patients access to existing technology, we cannot expect much saving from reducing this kind of quality.

The analytical question then is how to target for cuts those real program benefits whose absence would do the least damage. The objective is to find mechanisms that, in the quantity area, would reduce services of the least value per dollar spent and, in the quality area, would reduce amenities that have no clear effect on health (such as short waiting times for visits and freedom to choose high-cost providers). If such changes are successful, it may be possible to share some of the resulting cost savings with beneficiaries and—although we cannot be very optimistic about this—make them as well as taxpayers better off.

Insufficient State Discretionary Power

In contrast to the preceding problems, the issue of state control is related not to the outcome of the Medicaid program but rather to the process or institutional arrangements by which that outcome is reached. The fundamental presumption is that if the proper process or institutional arrangements were in place, a proper outcome would emerge.

The criticism is that there has been too much federal control over the process and too little power lodged at lower levels of government. If the decision-making process could be largely transferred from the federal government to state governments, the concrete problems of how much costs should be reduced and what form the cuts should take would generally be transferred to state governments. Federal concern would be limited to financing, to the size of federal transfers primarily, with only secondary concern about how those transfers are used, although the federal government might well play a role in research and assistance, helping states implement the plans that seem to be most successful in other areas. Although states would face many of the same tough trade-offs, the hope is that they could make choices better tailored to local circumstances and local preferences than the federal government.

This devolution of power to the states is a general approach to solving the Medicaid problem, and we discuss several possible variations in detail below. At one extreme, devolution could simply mean block grants, although there would still be the problem of how to determine the size of the grants. A more moderate variant would continue something like the present matching arrangements, but with much less restriction on state decisions concerning benefits, eligibility, and reimbursement. A third, even more limited form would remove just a few of the current restrictions. We consider each of these alternatives as well as others. A crucial element in our proposals for Medicaid reform is devolution of power to the lowest feasible level of decision as a method of controlling costs. The hope is that a more efficient structure for decision making will in fact lead to better decisions.

Notes

1. Eligibility for AFDC benefits requires that at least one parent be deceased, continually absent from the home, or physically or mentally incapacitated. In some states families with an unemployed father are also eligible.

2. For evidence of work response to cash transfers, see Harold Watts and Albert Rees, eds., *The New Jersey Income Maintenance Experiment*, vol. 2, *Labor Supply Responses* (New York: Academic Press, 1977); Robert Moffitt, "The Labor Supply Response in the Gary Income Maintenance Experiment," *Journal of Human Resources*, vol. 14, no. 4 (Fall 1979); Michael Keeley, Philip Robins, Robert Spiegelman, and Richard West, "The Labor Supply Effects and Costs of Alternative Negative Income Tax Programs," *Journal of Human Resources*, vol. 13, no. 1 (Winter 1978).

3. See table C–1, appendix C.

4. Congressional Budget Office, "Medicaid: Choices for 1982 and Beyond," June 1981. This happens, in part because of persons with variable incomes, who may have little or no income and receive Medicaid during part of the year but earn at a high rate for the rest of the year.

5. To measure eligibility standards in real terms, we must divide the states' income limit by a local price index. One measure of leniency in Medicaid eligibility, therefore, is the maximum allowed income for a four-person recipient family with dependent children as a fraction of the local cost of a lower budget for a four-person family—that is, the maximum share of a lower budget that a family could have and still be eligible for Medicaid. In 1978 this fraction ranged from 41 percent in New York City and 57 percent in Green Bay, Wisconsin, to 15 percent in Houston and 11 percent in Atlanta. Thus some persons receiving Medicaid in Wisconsin had real incomes over five times that of some persons with incomes too high to be served in Georgia.

6. For further evidence based on regression analysis, see Thomas Grannemann, "Reforming National Health Programs for the Poor," in Mark Pauly, ed., *National Health Insurance: What Now? What Later? What Never?* (Washington, D.C.: American Enterprise Institute, 1980).

7. *Statistical Abstract of the United States 1981*, 102d ed. (Washington, D.C., December 1981).

8. See Richard J. Cebula, Robert M. Kohn, and Richard K. Vedder, "Some Determinants of Interstate Migration of Blacks," *Western Economic Journal*, vol. 11, no. 4 (December 1973).

9. Grannemann, "Reforming National Health Programs," pp. 106–7.

4

Goals for a Reformed Medicaid Program

The Medicaid program was set up in haste. With the subsequent continued furor over national health insurance, there has been little opportunity for reflection on the appropriate objectives for Medicaid and the kinds of program alterations that might best achieve those objectives. This chapter of our study provides such reflection. One of the major difficulties in sorting things out is to separate changes that people wish could be made but that are impossible from those that are possible. But before confronting the question of feasibility, it is wise to define what we regard as desirable in principle—bearing in mind that in doing so we may be setting up competing goals, which may not be simultaneously attainable.

Externalities and Equity

Why do we have Medicaid at all? If the answer is "to help the poor," the standard rebuttal is that such a goal could be achieved better, and at lower administrative cost, by simple transfers of income, permitting the recipients to finance their medical care however they wish. At politically feasible transfer levels, the poor would surely not become well off under such an arrangement, but they would have somewhat more income, and it is likely that they would purchase some medical insurance. It is also likely that, in general, they would buy less extensive coverage than is provided implicitly in the Medicaid program and that some would not purchase any insurance at all.

The amount of medical care consumed would then almost certainly be below what it is now. Perhaps equally important, given current institutional arrangements and practices, many lower-income persons might obtain care and yet not pay for that care, returning the system to a kind of private, largely involuntary system in which the cost of care for nonpayers is borne by users who do pay. Of course, institutional arrangements could be changed so that hospitals and physicians would be encouraged to refuse care to those unwilling to pay. But if that happened or if lower-income individuals themselves voluntarily refrained from care, many taxpayers with somewhat higher incomes would probably be bothered by the thought that some poor people were going without medical care that could be of benefit in their illnesses. Medical care that is perceived to alleviate suffering in others is something many of us are willing to pay for. Moreover, medical care for the poor can be considered a "public good" in that the benefits of knowing that the poor have adequate medical care accrue to everyone.

This is one concrete manifestation of what economists have called an externality—that is, a situation in which use of services by one person benefits others. Many persons would benefit (feel better) if a sick person received beneficial medical care. Although some of the motive for this externality may be self-interest (if, for example, the sufferer had a contagious disease or would be more likely to be unable to work because of illness), it is probable that for many taxpayers there is a kind of altruistic demand for medical care for those likely to purchase little care on their own—who would probably be those with lower incomes. This specific motive with regard to medical care is more than a desire to raise the total income of low-income individuals. It manifests itself in the fear that, if just given spendable income, poor people might not spend enough of it on medical care.

This motive is sufficient to explain why taxpayers support a program like Medicaid and why it is politically viable. It is almost surely true in addition, however, that the desire to subsidize medical care varies among taxpayers. Some of the variation is probably related to what we might call the "taste" for altruism. But much is also due to differences in conventional determinants of demand, such as income and prices. Regardless of their source, variations in taxpayers' demands for Medicaid need to be considered in designing alternatives to the present form of the Medicaid program.

If a fully federal program were enacted, for example, it would almost surely require the same standards for benefits and eligibility everywhere in the country. But a single level of benefits would necessarily fail to take into account differences in taxpayers' demands in different areas. In particular, unless the federal program at least allowed for state supplementation, it would prevent taxpayers inclined to generosity above the average in some areas of the country from providing the additional benefits and increased eligibility they would like. Conversely, it would prevent taxpayers in other areas who, because of their relatively low incomes or preferences, would have preferred to spend more on other things from doing so. Geographical decentralization, in contrast, would permit groups with different

FIGURE 1
STATE DEMAND AND TOTAL
DEMAND FOR MEDICAID

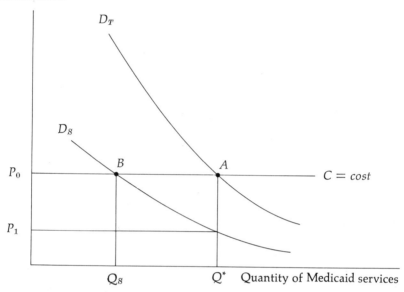

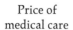

preferences to choose outcomes more in accord with those preferences. In a democracy an arrangement that permits government actions to approximate individual voters' desires more closely seems, almost by definition, to be preferable.

The catch here is that we cannot justifiably treat each state in isolation. The basic principle is straightforward. At any level of benefits or eligibility, we think of two quantities: first, the demand of taxpayers for Medicaid benefits within their own state and, second, the willingness of taxpayers in all other states to pay for additional benefits or eligibility for beneficiaries in that state. We want to push benefits or eligibility up until the sum of the marginal value of Medicaid to taxpayers, both in state and out of state, just equals the cost of increasing benefits or raising eligibility.

This situation can be represented graphically by means of demand curves. In figure 1, for example, D_S is the in-state demand, that is, the sum of valuations by state residents of Medicaid benefits for that state's poor population. We assume that the state's political process yields this as its demand schedule, at least approximately. To get a national demand for benefits in that state, we must add (vertically) the marginal valuations of persons in other states. This is represented by the total demand curve, D_T. The optimal level of benefits then would be at the quantity Q^* determined by the point where total demand (in-state plus out-of-state) intersects the curve representing the marginal cost of medical care.

This figure illustrates the rationale for a federal role in the provision of medical care to the poor. In the absence of federal assistance, the state would have to pay the full cost of medical services and would face an effective price of P_0. Given its in-state demand curve, it would choose a level of spending for medical care for the poor at Q_s. But this is clearly too little for an efficient allocation once the preferences of out-of-state individuals are taken into account. The state might, however, be induced to expand benefits to Q^* if the effective price of providing benefits were lowered to P_1 as a result of federal matching payments. The federal matching share that would be required is $(P_0 - P_1)/P_0$. Medicaid can thus be viewed as an attempt to encourage states to expand benefits to reflect the preferences of voters in other states for redistribution.

The question then is, Has the Medicaid program brought about the optimal level of Medicaid spending in all states? One suspects it has not. Although Medicaid's basic approach to solving the externality problem is sound, the parameters of the current matching-rate formula may not adequately reflect national demands given state responses to lower effective prices.

Although voter-taxpayers may have concern about the use of medical care by all poor people in the country, that concern may be stronger for the poor in their own state than for those in other states. The possibility of a geographic dimension of the externality is another important reason why there is a role for local governments. A crucial empirical question is whether or not voters *do* care more about medical care for the poor within their state's borders than about care for the poor in other states. Certainly, if the motivation for Medicaid is to curb contagious disease or to prevent debilitating illness that forces people into state and local welfare programs, the view that Medicaid externalities are local makes sense. One can also quote aphorisms about charity beginning at home and note that welfare programs, which are highly analogous, are state controlled. And the fact that we do not provide extensive medical services to the poor outside the United States despite their greater need is further evidence of some kind of geographic dimension in voter preferences. Medical care for the poor, it seems, has some characteristics of a local public good as well as of a national public good.

The public good approach thus provides the essential rationale for both federal and state involvement in Medicaid financing. A completely state run and financed program would not properly deal with cross-state externalities, and a wholly federal program would not properly adjust for voters' greater concern for the poor in their own area. Recognition of these simple principles allows us to make some fairly firm qualitative statements about the desirability of various possible forms of a federal-state program. We can, for example, describe what an ideal pattern of federal matching payments would be like. Potential applications are discussed in the next chapter.

In addition to adjusting for differences in voter-taxpayer preferences, a federal-state matching program may also permit more efficient handling of differences among states in medical care delivery systems. For one thing, the relative price of medical care in general varies across the country, and the optimal benefit package and eligibility standards should, therefore, vary with it—something that would be at best difficult to do under a fully federalized program but easier to do under a state-administered matching program. Somewhat surprisingly, higher medical care prices in an area can (as they should) lead to less restrictive eligibility standards, because the demand for Medicaid on the part of taxpayers is likely to be higher where high prices impede access to care.[1]

So far we have assumed that politicians and bureaucrats want to do what voters want, at least as they perceive the signals offered by majority rule. But this assumption is surely overoptimistic; the link between political decisions and voters' preferences can be weak. Bureaucracy has desires of its own, usually including the urge to spend more. At the federal level, it is difficult for voters to control those desires. The federal tax structure is quite productive of revenue, and voters have a hard time perceiving any alternatives to what the bureaucracy selects. With partial state financing, however, there are likely to be clearer signals and more effective constraints. If one state's bureaucracy pushes up the costliness of its program, the potential outflow of business and population and the inability to practice deficit financing without limit will act as a constraint. Paradoxically, the financial distress of the states may be not a problem but a desired outcome, since it is the fiscal manifestation of the process of curbing bureaucratic spending desires. Voters may rationally favor an institutional structure—partial state funding—that makes program expansion difficult and painful for politicians. The eagerness of state governors to shift the Medicaid program to the federal level, in other words, may be one of the best reasons to keep it where it is.

A final point about externalities is that, while concern for use of medical services by the poor provides a strong rationale for public intervention, that intervention need not take the precise form of current programs. As currently structured, the Medicaid program requires virtually complete public funding, and this feature may have discouraged states from expanding eligibility. An arrangement that required significant cost sharing from those able to pay but allowed more people to participate might better satisfy voter preferences for greater use of medical services by low-income groups. For recipients of cash transfers, the government may as well pay the full cost of care (except possibly for copayments designed to limit use of unnecessary services) and adjust cash payments accordingly. But for other low-income persons, limited public subsidies may be sufficient to induce purchase of medical insurance. In fact, persons with incomes lower than those of fully employed persons and above those of welfare recipients often have limited access to relatively low-cost group or employer health insurance plans, and they receive little benefit from medical tax deductions. Low rates of service use by such persons may therefore reflect higher than average effective prices of health insurance, which could be offset by partial public funding.

Horizontal Equity among Beneficiaries

Another possible objective for a reformed Medicaid program is greater equity among beneficiaries. Inequity in Medicaid may be broken down into two parts: categorical inequity and inequity among states. A family's eligibility depends on more than its income; it depends on whether it fits into certain categories. That is, eligibility depends on age, living arrangements, and the presence or absence of disability. Some of these characteristics, such as disability or blindness, may make sense as proxies for medical need. Others, as already noted, seem ultimately to be based on some notion of work effort response.

The second form of inequity involves variation in benefits or eligibility standards among states. Taxpayers in different states may differ in their valuation of Medicaid as they may differ in their demand for other public services. Perhaps the discomfort with the resulting benefit variation reflects an unexhausted cross-state externality—that is, a concern for the poor in other states that has not been adequately dealt with by current federal matching payments. If so, the solution is to design a federal response that alters state incentives so as to reflect more appropriately the preferences of voters in other states.

An additional rationale for a matching program is that, given the current federal tax structure, it may not be possible for voters to support the ideal arrangement at the federal level. The reason is that the level of Medicaid is chosen by majority rule, at least among representatives of the population. But there are surely some states whose representatives favor, and whose population would favor, higher than average levels of Medicaid at their current federal tax rates. A uniform benefit would leave the altruistic desires of these states unsatisfied. Of course, we could think of a federal arrangement in which their residents' federal taxes were raised to levels higher than those of other states' residents to pay for the extra Medicaid benefits they want, but this would be unconstitutional as well as politically unlikely. A more practical alternative would be to permit those taxpayers who want higher levels of Medicaid to have it, at least for their own states' poor, possibly with some matching.

Even if it should turn out that concern about use of medical care by the poor has no geographical dimension, at most that would only imply similar benefits in all states; but that is not inconsistent with a federal-state program. That is, in theory a federal-state program could always be as good as, and sometimes better than, a purely national program, making a strong case for retaining the federal-state nature of Medicaid. Such an observation does not, however, preclude making the structure of the program very different from its current form. In particular, current disparities in benefits among states may be too large, current federal regulation and control may be excessive, and it may be preferable to restructure the flow of federal funds to reduce, though probably not wholly to eliminate, such differences.

Equity among Taxpayers

As noted above, the burden on a taxpayer required to support a given level of Medicaid benefits depends on the state in which the taxpayer chooses to live. Those taxpayers who choose to live in a state with few poor people, with many taxpayers with high incomes, and with more commercial taxable property or income pay a smaller share of Medicaid program costs, other things being equal. Under a fully national (federalized) program, in contrast, their taxes would be the same regardless of their location.

If one regards Medicaid benefits as a kind of national public good, the inequity is obvious: different people pay different taxes for the same thing depending on the state in which they live, and this seems to violate a fundamental principle of horizontal equity. If, in contrast, one regards Medicaid benefits as a kind of local public good, then the case for equal tax burdens is not so clear. Having poor people as neighbors makes a taxpayer worse off because the more such people there are, the more taxes he or she must pay. But the same thing is true of other regional characteristics—the more snow there is, or the more pollution, or the more mosquitoes, or the higher the public sector wage scale, the higher taxes will have to be to achieve a given real public income—and it is not obvious that the federal government has any business trying to equalize "real public income." In many cases high taxes for Medicaid might be offset by other factors; for example, the cost of living tends to be lower in poor states. And taxes required to pay the state share of Medicaid costs are in any case only a tiny fraction (less than 1 percent) of the average taxpayer's income.

Business taxes also need to be considered. The same equity and location-efficiency issues raised in connection with equity for beneficiaries arise here. Suppose, for example, that the most efficient location for a new manufacturing plant is in a Snowbelt state with relatively large numbers of poor people and relatively generous benefits. Given current methods of taxing firms, the high taxes that accompany the location may cause the firm to select an alternative site, one less desirable from the viewpoint of production costs but with more than offsetting lower taxes. Yet the firm's departure from its optimal location will not change the total amount spent on Medicaid; it will only redistribute the burden to the other taxpayers in the state. In short, there is an inefficiency loss determined by the differences in real production costs and an inequity effect from the resulting disparities in the distribution of the tax burden. Similar comments apply to taxation and location of individuals. Here again we do not know how serious a quantitative problem this is; but in any case, appropriate adjustments in the federal matching percentage for the number of poor people in a state would help to offset it.

In addition to the problems of horizontal equity we have discussed, there may be a problem of vertical equity between taxpayers and recipients. This arises if low-income taxpayers feel the government is giving too many benefits, at their expense, to persons not very different from themselves. Because taxpayers in low-income states may resent giving benefits to a large share of the state's population, this problem of vertical equity could be a barrier to solving the problems of horizontal equity among states. In the end, it may force us to live with more inequality in tax burdens or benefits among states than high-income taxpayers might like.

To sum up: the primary forms of inequity associated with present financing of Medicaid are horizontal inequity among beneficiaries and among taxpayers. As we will show, alteration of the matching formula to take the number of poor persons and the state tax base into account would go a long way toward solving this problem for both groups, although perfect horizontal equity among both bene-ficiaries and taxpayers probably cannot be achieved with matching rates alone given the nature of taxpayers' demand for Medicaid and our imperfect knowledge of states' responses to matching rates.

Reduced Excess Burden

As noted above, some Medicaid payments go to people who are not really poor. This may offend our sense of equity. There are other reasons to be concerned about high levels of Medicaid eligi-bility. Running resources through the tax system has real and impor-tant economic costs. These costs are the excess burden or welfare cost of taxation, and they are far from trivial. "Excess burden" is a term used by economists to refer to the value of goods and ser-vices lost when taxation creates incentives for inefficient behavior by firms or workers. It represents the lost output, lost investment, and lost work effort brought about by high marginal tax rates. Recent estimates put the marginal welfare cost of federal taxation at about 20 percent, meaning that federally collected and expended tax dollars need to be 20 percent more productive than the private expenditures they displace to offset the extra cost of excess burden.[2] Of course, providing Medicaid to some "undeserving" persons is a necessary cost of ensuring that fewer of the poor slip through the safety net, but the critical point is that making the mesh of that net smaller costs money and costs real resources even beyond the Medicaid expendi-tures that show up in government budgets.

Efficiency in the Provision of Medical Care

The most serious kind of inefficiency related to Medicaid is likely to be that associated with the provision of medical care itself. There are three kinds of inefficiency here. First, in providing service to Medicaid beneficiaries and to others, hospitals and doctors might be able to use fewer inputs to produce the same output, with the same qualitative characteristics. This is the definition of what economists call technical inefficiency, and what politicians and the media call "fat": the idea that current input can be used to do more or, conversely, that current output can be produced with fewer inputs.

The second kind of inefficiency, often called input-price inefficiency, comes from using the wrong mixture of inputs (given their relative costs) to produce current outputs. A different mixture—more of those inputs that are more productive in relation to their cost and fewer of those that are less productive in relation to their costs—could reduce costs. This kind of inefficiency might occur, for example, if a hospital used too many registered nurses in relation to the number of licensed practical nurses and nurses' aides.

The third kind of inefficiency, "demand inefficiency," occurs if cost is being minimized (so that both technical and input-price efficiency are achieved) but output of either the wrong quantity or the wrong quality is being produced. The cost is minimized, but the value or benefit to the user of the output is less than that cost. An unnecessarily long recovery period in a hospital after surgery, for example, would constitute quantitative inefficiency. Using an expensive tertiary-care unit in a teaching hospital (with batteries of tests and procedures) for a common and simple surgical procedure or consuming an expensive emergency room visit for a minor problem would consitute qualitative inefficiency. Note that to detect either of these variants of "demand inefficiency" one must know more than just cost; one must know what things are worth to users. A laboratory test produced in the most efficient manner possible is still inefficient if the results that test yields are worth less than its cost. Note too that demand inefficiency is not limited to tests or procedures that are worthless; it also applies to those that may be of considerable objective value, but a value less than the cost.

"Fat" has not, from all the empirical evidence we have, been a major contributor to the inflation of hospital costs nor is there any large-sample evidence of special Medicaid "fat" once eligibility is established. There is no evidence that hospitals or doctors are producing the care they produce any more inefficiently or efficiently now than they did before Medicaid. Our ability to discover ways to squeeze out fat, and only fat, from the current system is therefore limited at best.

Rather, most empirical work points to a different conclusion. Virtually all the inflation in medical care cost per unit, in excess of that attributable to inflation in general, is due to more quantity and, especially, more quality, or style, in medical care. In other words, the *nature* of the product has been changed. And this change has not been worthless. Medical care is better now than it used to be, including medical care received by the poor. It is more effective; it is more humane; it is given in situations that better preserve human dignity. What we do not know is whether this extra quality, and the moderate amount of extra quantity that has accompanied it, are worth what they cost, either to the beneficiaries who use them or to the taxpayers who pay for them. As Medicaid has moved the poor into mainstream medicine, the stream has begun to flow faster and faster, but in a direction and in a way that no one is sure are appropriate, not just for the poor but for everyone.

Why have the style and quantity of medical care been increasing? In part, to be sure, it is because new and apparently better ways of treating patients have been discovered. But this technical change has been assisted and to a considerable extent caused by the high amount of insurance coverage. Moreover, higher costs appear to be traceable primarily not to new high-level technology but to the spread of well-known ordinary technology.

The reason for this result is simple: when insurance pays, the user of medical care is less deterred by financial cost than when the user pays. That is presumably the reason why poor people's use of physicians' services has increased; Medicaid will now pay. Insurance without copayments also encourages persons to select the best and often most expensive style of care available in their community. The term for the behavioral response to the presence of insurance is "moral hazard," and in the case of medical care it has both a quantitative and a qualitative manifestation.

Because medical insurance reduces the price to users of medical care below its cost, it induces the user to obtain units of quantity and quality that are worth less to him than they cost; it engenders demand inefficiency. Of course, it also provides benefits—reduction in risk and, for poor people, the use of units of care that, if they are not worth what they cost to the direct user, are worth something to the taxpayers who subsidize them.

The problem is that appropriate comparisons of costs and benefits are not automatically made under the current system of insurance, which includes Medicaid. The goal of reform, then, is to think of systems that permit the appropriate comparisons to be made. An even more important point, however, is this: whatever method of reform is chosen to reduce costs, some aspects of quality, access, or free choice will have to be sacrificed. It will not be possible in a practical way to cut costs for all beneficiaries without doing damage. The object then, as we have stated, is to think of ways that cut costs by eliminating the least marginally beneficial, that is, the least important, aspect of medical care for each beneficiary.

Notes

1. For evidence, see Thomas Grannemann, "Reforming National Health Programs for the Poor," in Mark Pauly, ed., *National Health Insurance: What Now? What Later? What Never?* (Washington, D.C.: American Enterprise Institute, 1980).

2. Edgar Browning and William Johnson, "Taxation and the Cost of National Health Insurance," in Pauly, *National Health Insurance*, pp. 31–51.

5

Federal-State Financing Relationships: A Catalog of Policy Options

This chapter briefly evaluates a number of alternative approaches to changing the Medicaid financing system. Some of the alternatives have been discussed as options by the Reagan administration or considered by Congress; others have been included here for their interesting properties or simply to represent the range of policy options available. We evaluate each alternative by its ability to improve recipient and taxpayer equity and satisfy voter preferences; we also consider the effectiveness of each device in controlling federal and total Medicaid costs. The alternatives have been ordered to the extent possible, starting with those that seem to be incapable of producing the desired outcomes and concluding with those that appear to be the most promising. Because the alternatives have been specified in general terms rather than as detailed plans, a wide range of outcomes are possible under any particular option, depending on its specific form and the chosen level of funding.

To evaluate the various options, we employ simulation based on a model of state behavior and empirically estimated price elasticities that measure states' responsiveness to changes in the federal matching rate. This approach differs from that used to make actuarial projections of Medicaid expenditures in both its objectives and its methods. We are not attempting to predict a specific value for future Medicaid expenditures; instead we are trying to determine how each policy option would alter outcomes in relation to what they would otherwise have been. Because our estimates account for the behavior of states in response to altered federal incentives, our results add a dimension missing from actuarial models and can, in fact, be used in conjunction with such models to make better predictions. In this study, however, we simply present our outcome measures as values relative to a base-line average or as percentage changes from current-law estimates.[1] It should also be recognized that there may be considerable imprecision in our estimates both because it is impossible for the model to take account of all possible factors influencing the behavior of state policy makers and because of the statistical imprecision of estimated price elasticities. In any case, our basic conclusions do not depend on the specific values of the elasticities; they require only some degree of responsiveness by states to price. Despite their limitations we believe the analysis and simulation results provide useful (and the best available) first-order predictions of outcomes under various policy alternatives.

Simple Block Grant

One much-discussed way to aid states is through basic block grants. Unlike matching rates, a block grant does not make an *increase* in Medicaid benefits cost the state any less than if the state paid the whole bill; it simply replaces "front end" state funding up to the level of the block grant.[2] What, then, would be the effect on the benefits provided in the various states of a switch from the current matching system to block grants?

The outcome depends on the size of the block grant; there are two basic cases. First, for block grants that are any less than the state would have spent with no federal help, states can be expected to provide roughly the same benefits as they would have chosen with no federal assistance. That is, states would supplement the federal grant only to the extent necessary to bring benefits up to where they would be without the grant. Replacing current matching funds with small block grants would therefore tend to move states back toward their pre-Medicaid levels of medical care for the poor (adjusted for changes in income and prices since 1966). Besides drastically reducing benefits throughout the country, such a step would aggravate inequality among recipients, since those levels were even less uniform than the current ones.

In the second case—for a block grant larger than what the state would spend without federal help—we would not expect the state to augment the grant with state funds; there would be no price-reducing effect of matching to induce it to do so. In other words, without matching at the margin, any extra Medicaid benefits would cost the state 100 percent of actual cost and, since the state was not willing to pay the full cost of such benefits before the block grant, there is no reason (except for a small income effect) for the state to provide such benefits when federal block grant dollars can be substituted for front-end state spending.[3] In this situation—with state Medicaid spending determined by and equal to the amount of the block grant— financing of Medicaid would, in effect, be wholly federalized, with state responsibilities limited to administration. This might be an

TABLE 9

ELASTICITIES OF STATE DEMAND FOR MEDICAID

	Price Elasticity	Income Elasticity
Total Medicaid	−0.78	1.23
AFDC child recipients	−0.30	2.17
AFDC adult recipients	−0.25	2.32
AFDC child benefit level	−0.26	0.26
AFDC adult benefit level	−0.29	0.61

SOURCE: Thomas W. Grannemann, "Reforming National Health Programs for the Poor," in Mark Pauly, ed., *National Health Insurance: What Now? What Later? What Never?* (Washington, D.C.: American Enterprise Institute, 1980).

acceptable option if we thought the federal government had the information to determine the optimal level of benefits in each state and was willing to provide block grants for the full amount of Medicaid expenditures.[4] But if the level the federal government chose as optimal were anywhere near or greater than current average benefits, such a plan would require an enormous increase in federal expenditures. To summarize, because block grants remove the incentive for states to provide higher benefits, maintaining Medicaid benefits near current levels with block grants would require much greater federal spending.

How would a switch to block grants from the current matching system affect the benefits provided in various states? The outcome in each state would depend on its current matching rate and hence its per capita income. Suppose the plan was to keep federal spending at current levels in each state. If a block grant plan were adopted, a high-income state that currently receives a 50 percent matching rate would face a 100 percent increase in the effective marginal price of providing care (the change from paying 50 percent to 100 percent of the cost of any extra benefits). What would be the effect of this price increase? A recent study by Grannemann estimates the response of states to changes in the federal matching rate. In that study the effects of determinants of state Medicaid expenditures, eligibility, and benefits were investigated through a voter-choice model of state behavior. Statistically significant responses of Medicaid spending were found to both the federal matching rate and taxpayers' income and to other factors. Estimated elasticities—that is, the percentage change in real Medicaid benefits in response to a 1 percent change in the state taxpayer price or income—are shown in table 9.[5]

TABLE 10

Simulated Effects of Block Grants at Current Level of Federal Funding, Representative States

| State | Relative Real Benefits[a] | | Percentage Change in Benefits |
	Initial	Simulated	
California	89	44	−50
Georgia	69	46	−34
Illinois	99	50	−50
Mississippi	57	44	−23
New York	210	107	−49
Pennsylvania	107	61	−43
Texas	60	34	−44
Wisconsin	232	135	−42

a. Dollar Medicaid payments per person below the poverty level adjusted for interstate differences in medical care prices as a percentage of initial U.S. average benefits per poor person.

As indicated there, the elasticity of the number of child beneficiaries with respect to the state's effective price is about −0.30, and the elasticity of benefits per recipient is −0.26. These estimates suggest that providing a high-income state with a block grant (which constitutes a 100 percent increase in price) would produce about a 30 percent reduction in the number of recipients and a 26 percent reduction in benefits per recipient. A low-income state that started with a 75 percent matching rate would have its effective marginal price increased 300 percent, from 25 percent to 100 percent of cost, by a switch to block grants. This price effect would provide an even greater incentive for reductions in number of recipients and benefits per recipient. In this example we would expect total spending to fall to a lower bound determined by the level of the federal grant itself, which in this low-income state is 75 percent of current total spending. With such a large incentive to reduce benefits, we would surely not expect low-income states to supplement a federal block grant of this size.

Using the previously estimated overall price elasticity of −0.78, we simulated a shift to block grants, assuming that each state was provided a grant equal to the amount of the federal matching funds it now receives. No state is expected to supplement the federal grant after allowing time for full response by the state to the higher effective price of Medicaid. Table 10 shows the simulated effect on real benefits in a few representative states. Here and in later simulations we employ a measure of real Medicaid benefits per person below the poverty level that is adjusted for interstate differences in medical care prices.[6] A relative real benefit of 100 would equal the U.S. average before any change. In all states in the simulation, state spending falls to zero, and the level of spending is determined wholly by the federal grant. Wide variations in benefits among states remain with their adverse implications for horizontal equity.

Although we cannot know how long adjustment to such a change would take and the block grant itself sets a floor to spending cuts, these calculations do nevertheless indicate the direction and potentially large magnitude of long-run responses by states to block grants. If federal matching funds were replaced by block grants of comparable size, low-income states would make large cuts in benefits and would probably choose not to supplement the federal grant with their own funds. High-income states would also cut back benefits significantly, probably by an even higher percentage since the federal block grant would replace a smaller fraction of their current program expenditures. Of course, it is possible that states would choose to supplement the grant—particularly in the near term—but it is quite unlikely that in the long run they would maintain benefits anywhere near their current levels. In summary, a simple block grant plan with grants roughly equal to current federal payments would almost certainly cause severe reductions in Medicaid expenditures and could also lock in the present interregional inequities in the distribution of federal funds. To keep benefits from falling, the block grant would have to equal at least the sum of current federal and state spending. Future programs should not be designed with the expectation that states would do much to supplement block grants for Medicaid.

Cap on Federal Expenditures

In 1981 the Reagan administration unsuccessfully advocated a plan for capping federal Medicaid expenditures by limiting federal payments to states under the current matching formula. Unlike the reduction in the rate of federal matching that was adopted in the 1981 Budget Reconciliation Act, this plan proposed an absolute limit on federal payments. The increase in federal payments was to be no greater than the overall inflation rate, requiring states to cover 100 percent of the cost of any real increase in Medicaid expenditures. Each state would have received the current federal matching share for amounts of real benefits up to the level of those currently provided. This would produce a discontinuity in the states' effective price schedule for Medicaid—one price set by matching rates for amounts less than or equal to current benefits and a second price equal to 100 percent of costs for any increase above that amount.

What would the effect of such a cap be? In the absence of any shift in demand, states would be expected to maintain their current Medicaid spending. But this method of limiting federal expenditures would seriously inhibit states from expanding benefits if voters' demand for Medicaid increased, say, in response to growth in state population or income. And the disincentives for expansion would be greater for low-income states than for high-income states. A low-income state with a 75 percent matching rate, for example, would have its effective price for expansions in Medicaid benefits quadrupled, from 25 percent to 100 percent of costs, while a high-income state would face only a doubling of the effective price, from 50 to 100 percent of costs. Thus low-income states would require a greater shift in demand to overcome the notch in the effective price schedule. Even if income in the low-income state expanded to that of the high-income state, benefits would be unlikely to rise to equality because the cap would eliminate the federal incentive for such an expansion. The original high-income states would thus maintain their favored treatment and higher benefits.

The price and income elasticities shown in table 9 can be used to obtain a rough estimate of the increase in income required for a state to overcome the notch and begin expanding benefits. The aggregate price elasticity is −0.78 for all recipients combined, and the aggregate income elasticity is 1.23. The percentage change in state per capita income required to overcome a cap-induced rise in marginal price would be e_p/e_y, or 63 percent (−0.78/1.23) of the change in marginal price. A low-income state, which would face a 300 percent increase in the effective marginal price of Medicaid, would require a 190 percent increase in real income before it would expand benefits *at all*. The comparable figure for the high-income state with a 50 percent matching rate, and therefore facing a 100 percent price increase, is 63 percent. These numbers are sufficient to show that a cap on federal expenditures would effectively freeze all state Medicaid programs at their current levels in real terms, an effect that would not be overcome by moderate changes in state demand.

Would it be desirable to have such a freeze? A cap would lock in the inequitable distribution of federal dollars and, in the long run, would hurt most the low-income, but growing, Sunbelt states that now have low benefits but might otherwise be expected to expand them as their fiscal capacity increases. Without the availability of additional federal matching dollars, such states would probably never catch up with higher-income states in Medicaid benefits or federal assistance, even if income differences narrowed substantially. Such a plan would also injure states with rapidly growing elderly populations. In summary, a strict cap on federal Medicaid payments might control federal spending in the short run, but it would certainly not be a permanent solution to the problems of Medicaid, precisely because it would freeze in current inequities and inefficiencies.

Across-the-Board Uniform Reduction in Matching Rates

A reduction in federal matching payments to states of up to 4.5 percent by fiscal year 1984 was enacted into law as part of the Omnibus Budget Reconciliation Act of 1981. This plan appears to treat all states equally (ignoring the special conditions under which states might avoid part of the cut). But in fact it does not do so because the equal percentage-point reduction applies to a larger federal percentage for low-income states. Low-income states, therefore, face a greater percentage increase in the effective price to the state taxpayer of providing Medicaid benefits. For example, a state with a matching rate of F currently faces an effective price of $(1 - F)C$, where C is the local cost of a standardized unit of medical care. With a 4.5 percent reduction in federal matching payments, the effective price becomes $(1 - 0.955F)C$. For a high-income state starting with a 50 percent matching rate, the effective price rises from $0.5C$ to $0.5225C$—a 4.5 percent increase. But for a lower-income state, starting with a 75 percent matching rate, the effective price rises from $0.25C$ to $0.2838C$—a 13.5 percent increase.

The "uniform" cut therefore gives low-income states a greater incentive to cut back Medicaid benefits than high-income states. Using the estimated price elasticity of -0.78, we calculate that the low-income state of our example would be expected to reduce real Medicaid benefits by 10.5 percent and the high-income state by 3.5 percent. Given the current imbalance in benefits between high-income and low-income states, this is exactly the opposite of what one would desire to improve equity among recipients.

We simulated a 4.5 percent reduction in federal matching payments. The results for representative states are presented in table 11. Note that the expected percentage reduction in real benefits in the two relatively low-income states, Mississippi and Georgia, is much larger than in the other representative states. Aggregating the simulated effects in all states, we find that the 4.5 percent reduction is estimated to reduce total federal payments by 9 percent in the long run because of state benefit reductions induced by the higher effective

48

TABLE 11

Simulated Effects of 4.5 Percent Across-the-Board Reduction in Matching Rates, Representative States

State	Matching Rate		Relative Real Benefits[a]		Percentage Change in Benefits	State Tax Burden[b]		Percentage Change in Tax Burden
	Initial[c]	Simulated	Initial	Simulated		Initial	Simulated	
California	50.00	47.75	89	86	−3.5	0.72	0.73	0.8
Georgia	66.28	63.30	69	65	−6.9	0.47	0.48	1.3
Illinois	50.00	47.75	99	96	−3.5	0.66	0.67	0.8
Mississippi	77.36	73.88	57	50	−12.0	0.40	0.41	1.6
New York	50.88	48.59	210	202	−3.6	1.74	1.75	0.9
Pennsylvania	56.78	54.22	107	102	−4.6	0.57	0.57	1.0
Texas	55.75	53.24	60	58	−4.4	0.42	0.43	1.0
Wisconsin	58.02	55.41	232	221	−4.9	0.88	0.89	1.1

a. Dollar Medicaid payments per person below the poverty level adjusted for interstate differences in medical care prices as a percentage of initial U.S. average benefits per poor person.

b. State Medicaid payments as a percentage of aggregate adjusted gross income on individual income tax returns.

c. Rate before the 1981 Reconciliation Act.

49

TABLE 12
SIMULATED EFFECTS OF 40 PERCENT MINIMUM MATCHING RATES, AFFECTED STATES

State	Relative Real Benefits[a]		Percentage Change in Benefits
	Initial	Simulated	
Alaska	52	44	−15.6
California	89	76	−14.7
Connecticut	146	123	−15.6
Illinois	99	92	−7.7
Nevada	59	52	−11.1
New Jersey	139	119	−14.4
Washington	90	86	−4.3
Wyoming	48	41	−14.0

a. Dollar Medicaid payments per person below the poverty level adjusted for interstate differences in medical care prices as a percentage of initial U.S. average benefits per poor person.

marginal price of Medicaid as well as the direct reduction in federal matching payments.

Reduction of the Minimum Matching Rate

Another proposal, considered by Congress in 1981 but rejected, was to reduce the minimum federal matching share from 50 percent to 40 percent. In theory, this plan would have reduced the federal contribution only to some high-income states and thereby encouraged cuts in benefits in some states where they currently tend to be high. The proposed reduction in matching rates would have increased the effective price of Medicaid to the states most affected from 0.5C to 0.6C, or by 20 percent, but it would not have affected benefits in states with higher federal matching shares.[7] The overall Medicaid price elasticity of −0.78 indicates that this plan, allowing sufficient time for adjustment, would induce those states to reduce real Medicaid expenditures by up to 16 percent. Some states would be affected less since the matching rate would not drop all the way to 40 percent, and many states would not have their rates changed at all.

Table 12 shows the current Medicaid benefits per person below the poverty level and the forecasted new benefits as percentages of the current average U.S. benefits for states affected by this change. The group of affected states includes more states with real benefits below the national average than states with above-average benefits, suggesting that in practice the method would not focus Medicaid cuts where they would do the least harm. We would expect this plan to reduce federal expenditures by about 6 percent and leave total state payments virtually unchanged after expected reductions in quantities of services provided.

Full Federalization

Perhaps the most obvious way to achieve equity among recipients and taxpayers would be to change Medicaid into a federal program with uniform national benefits and eligibility criteria financed through the federal tax system. An equitable federal program would be more difficult to design, however, than one might at first perceive. Medical care prices and living costs vary greatly among states and localities, and both eligibility criteria and benefits would need to be adjusted to reflect these differences. In addition, under a uniform national plan it would not be possible for states to tailor the program to local needs, preferences, and prices. As a result, nonoptimal levels of aggregate Medicaid spending would probably be selected. If preferences for Medicaid are local, the levels might well be lower than optimal in many areas since taxpayer-donors could not ensure that extra benefits would go to the poor in their local area and might therefore desire to spend less. This problem could be alleviated by allowing states to supplement the federal benefits, but that would violate the objective of equity among recipients and lead to duplicative administrative expenses.

Under most of the federal-state plans discussed in the preceding sections, states could be free to determine whether funds are used for additional recipients or for higher benefits. This flexibility would not be possible in a uniform federal program. Such an outcome might be viewed as desirable by persons primarily or exclusively concerned with equal treatment of the poor among states and within states. But an efficient allocation of resources would call for different distributions of benefits in different areas. For example, in areas with high medical care costs it might be more efficient to substitute other services for medical care and have slightly lower real Medicaid benefits. In such high-cost areas voters might rationally favor less stringent eligibility criteria because the high cost impedes access of needy persons with somewhat higher incomes to a greater degree. Thus, even within a given Medicaid budget, we might prefer resources to be skewed toward extra recipients at the expense of extra services in high-cost areas.

Differences in the relative prices of individual services should also enter into the determination of Medicaid benefits. In rural states nursing home care may be relatively inexpensive but home care services more costly to deliver. This suggests that on efficiency grounds interstate differences should be allowed in the mixture of institutional and noninstitutional services for the elderly. With a uniform federal program, it would be difficult to make the necessary adjustments.

In summary, a federal program may be the only way to guarantee equal treatment for all poor persons in the United States. So, for those who place extremely high priority on equity for individual recipients over the competing goal of efficiency, federalization may be the preferred option. Much-improved if not perfect equity among recipients, however, is possible under a variety of options; federalization is not the only solution. It would be possible, for example, to come much closer than we now are to full equity among recipients by adjusting matching rates. Alternatively, we could ensure equality of Medicaid spending per poor person under an appropriate block grant scheme, such as the one we consider below.

Objective-Oriented Matching Rates

Another approach is to attempt to manipulate federal matching rates to achieve some specified distribution of benefits and tax burdens among states. For purposes of evaluating outcomes, we define three specific objectives, in precise and admittedly somewhat overrestrictive terms for simplicity:

- Recipient equity—total real Medicaid benefits per poor person are the same in every state.
- Taxpayer equity—state Medicaid expenditures as a share of state taxpayer income are the same in every state.
- Voter demand satisfaction—states are free to determine their own Medicaid expenditures in response to federal matching payment incentives.

It is not generally possible to find a set of matching rates that fully satisfy all three objectives of recipient equity, taxpayer equity, and voter demand satisfaction as we have defined them.[8] When states determine Medicaid expenditures in response to federal matching, if we set matching rates to equalize benefits per poor person, state tax burdens will differ; and if we set matching rates to equalize tax burdens, variation in benefits will remain. It is possible, however, to achieve these goals in part. First, it is possible to find changes that bring about improvements by all three criteria, even if they are not all perfectly satisfied. Second, it is possible to find matching rates that satisfy any two of these objectives provided appropriate information is available and, in some cases, the policy maker is willing to impose certain constraints on the states.

Complete Recipient Equity and Complete Taxpayer Equity. If one assumes (perhaps unrealistically) that federal policy makers can make a reasonable guess at the optimal level of Medicaid benefits per poor person and if states are willing to forgo the freedom to determine their Medicaid benefits, then it is possible to find matching rates that satisfy both recipient equity and taxpayer equity. First, a uniform benefit level and an effective state tax rate (share of the state taxpayers' income to be used for Medicaid) are set by the federal government. To produce these uniform benefits and tax burdens in every state, the federal share of costs must be negatively related to the state's aggregate taxpayer income (or some other measure of fiscal capacity) and directly related to the number of poor and the cost of medical care in the state. The matching rates would also depend on how generous the standard benefits were and how large a state tax share was selected by federal policy makers. With this option, one could satisfy both recipient equity and taxpayer equity, but because states do not select the level of benefits, the voter demand satisfaction condition would not be met.

Approximate Recipient Equity with Perfect Demand Satisfaction. The second objective-oriented approach is designed to attain recipient equity and demand satisfaction. If one knows the state demand curves for Medicaid, it is possible to find a set of matching rates that would induce states to provide a desired level of benefits. To do this one needs to know the variables that affect state demand for Medicaid; the most important determinants of Medicaid spending have been identified elsewhere.[9]

Although such appropriately designed matching rates should on average induce the states to provide the desired aggregate amount of benefits, they would not necessarily result in any particular distribution of benefits among recipients. Because the factors that affect state demand for the number of recipients differ from those that affect the desired benefit level per recipient, it is not generally possible to find a single matching rate that will cause the state both to select a specified level of benefits and to serve a particular number of Medicaid recipients. We have argued, however, that such precision in satisfying federal desires is generally not desirable anyway. We can also expect state benefits to vary in practice because of factors not accounted for in the demand function used to compute matching rates. Such variations could be large. Random disturbances in the state decision-making process will also cause deviations from the norm.

Table 13 shows for selected states how rates might be changed and the predicted effect on benefits per poor person and on the burden on taxpayers. In many states the new matching rates would move both benefits and tax burdens closer to national means, producing improvements in both recipient and taxpayer equity. This would be true in New York, for example, where the plan would offer substantial savings for state taxpayers provided the simulated reduction in benefits occurred. In many low-benefit states, however, the higher matching rates would mean a reduced tax burden where taxpayers already spend less than the national average share of income on Medicaid benefits. This illustrates the competing nature of recipient equity and taxpayer equity with simple matching rates. This approach produces outcomes that satisfy voter preferences and equalize benefits for recipients (at least to the extent that we can predict state responses), but it still leaves variation among states in taxpayer equity as measured by the share of aggregate state income going to pay the state share of Medicaid expenses. If some variation in tax burdens was considered tolerable—and, because the share of taxpayers' income going to Medicaid is small, it might be—this approach would be attractive.

Improved Recipient Equity and Taxpayer Equity. A compromise between these two options would be to select a set of matching rates that achieve more taxpayer equity by sacrificing some degree of recipient equity. Since our ability to determine the optimal level of benefits is imprecise anyway and since such a plan might improve both recipient and taxpayer equity, altering the relationship of matching rates to income and linking them to the number of poor people in the state and aggregate taxpayer income might be an administratively simple way to improve the current system. Such alterations would reduce federal matching rates in high-income states that have relatively few poor persons but relatively well off taxpayers. This approach might be favored as a temporary remedy for the problem of recipient equity while we await more fundamental reforms.

Adding a Lump-Sum State Contribution. The inconsistency among the three goals—recipient equity, taxpayer equity, and demand satisfaction—in a matching system derives from the desire to control too many outcomes with too few policy parameters. That is, with just

TABLE 13

Simulated Effects of Matching Rates to Equalize Real Benefits at the U.S. Average, Representative States

State	Matching Rate		Relative Real Benefits[a]		Percentage Change in Benefits	State Tax Burden[b]		Percentage Change in Tax Burden
	Initial[c]	Simulated	Initial	Simulated		Initial	Simulated	
California	50.00	54.83	89	100	12	0.72	0.73	2
Georgia	66.28	77.84	69	100	44	0.47	0.45	−5
Illinois	50.00	50.30	99	100	1	0.66	0.66	0+
Mississippi	77.36	90.82	57	100	76	0.40	0.29	−29
New York	50.88	30.80	210	100	−52	1.74	1.16	−33
Pennsylvania	56.78	54.45	107	100	−7	0.57	0.56	−2
Texas	55.75	78.47	60	100	66	0.42	0.34	−19
Wisconsin	58.02	39.36	232	100	−57	0.88	0.55	−38

a. Dollar Medicaid payments per person below the poverty level adjusted for interstate differences in medical care prices as a percentage of initial U.S. average benefits per poor person.

b. State Medicaid payments as a percentage of aggregate adjusted gross income on individual income tax returns.

c. Rate before the 1981 Reconciliation Act.

one matching rate for a state, it is not possible both to induce the state to set benefits at a specified level and to have the state tax burden come out at the national average. But if we introduce another controlling feature in the form of a mandatory lump-sum state contribution selected for each state to equalize tax burdens, all three goals can, theoretically at least, be achieved simultaneously. If this approach were adopted, matching rates that determine the effective price to the state of providing additional Medicaid benefits would be set to induce approximately equal spending per poor person in each state. The lump-sum state contribution to program costs would be determined by a formula under which the payment would be larger for states the greater their aggregate taxpayer income or some other measure of state fiscal capacity. The state contribution would also be larger for states with higher federal matching percentages, but would be lower in states with many poor persons or high medical care prices.[10] One potential problem with such a plan is that states might view the state contribution as too high and choose to opt out of the Medicaid program altogether. There is some evidence from past and current spending behavior, however, that states would be willing to pay fairly substantial lump sums before turning down federal matching completely.

Block Grant with a Mandatory State Contribution

Another possible structure for a revised Medicaid program would make federal block grants to the states conditional on a specified state contribution to the program. The total expenditures—federal grant plus mandatory state contribution—could be made a function of the number of poor people, local medical care prices, and the local cost of living to ensure a uniform average real benefit per poor person below a specified fraction of the poverty level.

Under this plan the states would determine how benefits would be distributed among the poor, they would be free to develop their own cost-saving strategies, and they could use any savings to expand either benefits or the number of recipients or both. The size of the required state contribution could be set to equalize the burden on taxpayers among states. States could spend more if they wished, but without additional federal assistance. This would be an efficient solution to the externality problem only if (perhaps implausibly) there were absolutely no out-of-state voters' demand for spending beyond the uniform level and no geographical dimension in taxpayers' concern for the poor. Nevertheless, this plan is a means of achieving an equitable distribution of benefits while allowing for decentralized

TABLE 14

Simulated Effects of Block Grants with Mandatory State Contributions, Representative States

State	Relative Real Benefits[a]		Percentage Change in Benefits	State Tax Burden[b]		Percentage Change in Tax Burden
	Initial	Simulated		Initial	Simulated	
California	89	100	12	0.72	0.66	−9
Georgia	69	100	44	0.47	0.66	39
Illinois	99	100	1	0.66	0.66	−1
Mississippi	57	100	76	0.40	0.66	64
New York	210	100	−52	1.74	0.66	−62
Pennsylvania	107	100	−7	0.57	0.66	16
Texas	60	100	66	0.42	0.66	55
Wisconsin	232	100	−57	0.88	0.66	−25

a. Dollar Medicaid payments per person below the poverty level adjusted for interstate differences in medical care prices as a percentage of initial U.S. average benefits per poor person.

b. State Medicaid payments as a percentage of aggregate adjusted gross income on individual income tax returns.

state administration. It might, therefore, be the preferred option of those who dislike the centralized administration implied by federalization but also are uncomfortable with the disparities in benefits that accompany most matching arrangements. The basic plan could be modified to permit states to supplement the minimum spending level—thus allowing adjustment for local preferences and appealing to those who believe the federal role is to ensure a certain minimum rather than equal Medicaid spending among states.

The simulated outcomes of this approach for several states are presented in table 14. Note that both real benefits per poor person and the state tax burden are uniform among the states. At the level of benefits specified in this simulation, both federal and state Medicaid payments would remain about the same. Of course, spending could be modified to permit either cost savings or expansion of benefits.

This option for Medicaid financing is particularly appealing for several reasons. First, it ensures a minimum level of real benefits per poor person in every state. Second, it ensures an equitable distribution of the tax burden among states. Third, it permits states to supplement benefits at their own expense where state demands and local externalities suggest a need for extra benefits.[11] Since any supplementation could take place within the state administrative structure, this plan avoids the administrative problems and duplication that would arise in a federalized program if states decided to develop their own programs to supplement federal benefits. Fourth, unlike optimal-matching-rate formulas, this plan does not require detailed knowledge of state demand for Medicaid. Fifth, because states pay part of the costs, it does not require 100 percent federal funding to achieve an optimal level of benefits as conventional block grants do. Finally, it allows states to develop plans that reflect local needs, preferences, and relative prices. This approach of block grants with mandatory state contributions, perhaps with the addition of some federal matching at the margin, deserves particular consideration by policy makers.

Declining Matching Rates

Our most preferred form of federal-state financing is based on declining matching rates. Theoretically this approach can produce an optimal level of benefits in every state. Although there are some practical limitations, we first describe the theoretically preferred form of such a plan before outlining a more realistic approach that approximates the optimal one.

The matching-rate schemes discussed above all require that federal policy makers have considerable knowledge of state demands for Medicaid to determine and achieve an optimal benefit level. But even if federal policy makers cannot accurately estimate state demands, it may still be possible to find matching rates to promote optimal benefits. Even if preference for Medicaid has a geographical dimension, so that people care more about the poor in their own state, policy makers can estimate the out-of-state or "federal" demand for Medicaid—that is, the sum of the marginal valuation of voters outside the state. The trick is to structure the matching-rate formula so that it reflects the willingness of out-of-state taxpayers to pay for Medicaid; then the states' choice of benefits, given the specified matching-rate formula, will be optimal.

Figure 2 shows state demand, D_S, and out-of-state demand, D_N, for Medicaid benefits in a particular state, S. The total of these, D_T, determines the optimal level of benefits, Q^*—that is, where total demand equals marginal cost. Suppose federal policy makers can observe or otherwise determine out-of-state demand, D_N, but not D_S or D_T. Since the willingness to pay for extra benefits should decline as benefits increase, matching rates should also decline as Medicaid

FIGURE 2
DEMAND FOR MEDICAID AND EFFECTIVE PRICE SCHEDULE
WITH DECLINING MATCHING RATES

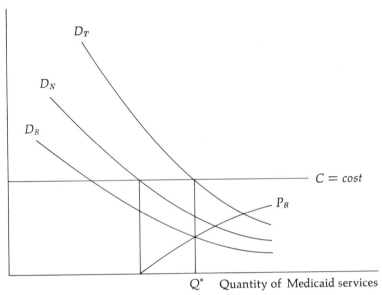

spending in a state is increased. Matching rates could be set to reflect the value of D_N at every level of benefits, Q. For all points to the left of the intersection of D_N with the marginal cost curve, the out-of-state demand alone exceeds the cost, and the federal government would pay 100 percent. Then the marginal matching rate (the rate applied to increments in expenditure) would begin to decline with Q. At the point where out-of-state marginal valuations sum to ⅔ of the cost, the matching rate would be ⅔, and so on. The effective marginal price to the state would be $P_S = 1 - F(Q)$, where the matching rate is an appropriate function of the aggregate state Medicaid benefits. That is, the amount the federal government would contribute for additional benefits would decline as benefits increased. In figure 2 this is shown by a rising curve, P_S, which represents the effective price of Medicaid to the state. The state would select the level of benefits where the price it faces, P_S, equals its demand; that would be at the optimal level, Q^*.

59

With an appropriate matching-rate structure of this type, the state should choose to provide optimal benefits regardless of local preferences for Medicaid within the state. This approach to matching rates does not necessarily produce equity for taxpayers; however, it may be possible to bring about greater taxpayer equity by adjusting inframarginal matching rates (ones that affect no state's decision) or by requiring a state contribution.

Because we do not have enough information on out-of-state demand for Medicaid to calculate precisely an optimal declining-matching-rate schedule, a more practical alternative is to define a schedule thought to approximate the optimal one. A simple version would have the matching rate decrease linearly with state expenditure over some range, with full federal funding below the range and full state funding above it. Another possibility along these lines would be to have matching decline in steps—for example, 100 percent federal funding to some minimum expenditure per poor person, then 75 percent federal expenditures up to 110 percent of the minimum, and so on, with no federal matching beyond some larger percentage of the minimum.

We simulated an application of the declining-rate approach by employing a linear declining-matching-rate formula in which matching rates decrease as benefits per poor person increase. The particular matching plan we simulated was designed so that at the margin the federal government paid full cost up to the level where the state's real benefits per poor person (payments adjusted for price differences) equaled 80 percent of the current U.S. average. Then matching decreased in proportion to the amount of spending down to zero at the point at which benefits equaled 120 percent of the current U.S. average. The lower limit effectively set a floor on benefits, so that benefits per poor person in each state would be at least 80 percent of the current U.S. average. The upper limit meant that states must pay the full cost of any benefits beyond 120 percent of the U.S. average.[12]

The matching rates are structured so that for a given level of state expenditures, M, rates are higher the greater the number of poor and the higher medical care prices in the state.[13] But the formula is also designed to compensate for interstate differences in medical care prices and number of poor people so that states with the same real benefits per poor person would have the same matching rate.

The simulation also allowed for a lump-sum contribution by each state.[14] The contribution is set so that, if the state chose to provide real benefits per poor person at the U.S. average, total state payments —matching share plus lump-sum contribution—as a share of state taxpayers' income would equal the U.S. average.[15] Thus states that

TABLE 15

Simulated Effects of Linearly Declining Matching Rates with Lump-Sum State Contributions, Representative States

State	Relative Real Benefits[a]		Percentage Change in Benefits	State Tax Burden[b]		Percentage Change in Tax Burden
	Initial	Simulated		Initial	Simulated	
California	89	98	10	0.72	0.64	−11
Georgia	69	89	27	0.47	0.57	21
Illinois	99	100	1	0.66	0.65	−2
Mississippi	57	84	47	0.40	0.50	25
New York	210	111	−47	1.74	0.78	−55
Pennsylvania	107	99	−8	0.57	0.65	15
Texas	60	87	45	0.42	0.59	39
Wisconsin	232	108	−53	0.88	0.70	−20

a. Dollar Medicaid payments per person below the poverty level adjusted for interstate differences in medical care prices as a percentage of initial U.S. average benefits per poor person.

b. State Medicaid payments as a percentage of aggregate adjusted gross income on individual income tax returns.

chose to provide above-average benefits would spend a greater than average share of their taxpayers' income on Medicaid.

The results of the simulation using this declining-matching-rate formula are presented in table 15. In nearly all states the new matching rates would move benefits toward the national average, the largest changes occurring in states with the most extreme levels of benefits. The plan thus clearly moves in the direction of improved recipient equity. Taxpayer equity would be improved as well, state tax burdens generally increasing where they had been low and decreasing where they had previously been high.

A declining-matching-rate formula would give states more freedom to determine benefits than the preceding option of block grants with state contributions. Still, by specifying the bounds of the matching range, federal policy makers could determine the range of state responses, because no state would choose to provide less than the minimum benefits if the federal government paid the full marginal cost of those services and because our estimates show that in the long run it would be unlikely for states to be willing to pay the full cost of benefits very far above the national average.

If this financing plan is implemented, federal policy makers could

easily vary the formula parameters to reflect current political preferences for higher or lower benefits and for either more or less cross-
state equality in benefits and taxes. With this declining-rate approach
the disparities in state benefits could be reduced gradually over a
number of years to ease the pain for high-benefit states by giving them
time to implement cost-saving measures. This could be done by
initially setting a wide range for matching, with some matching
allowed up to, say, 160 percent of the current U.S. average real benefit and down to 40 percent of the average. Over time the range could
be narrowed, according to an established schedule, perhaps to the
80–120 percent range of our simulation example or an even smaller
range if desired.

High-benefit states would still have the option of keeping their
benefits near current levels with some federal assistance at the margin
for amounts within the range; for amounts above the matching range,
states could provide benefits at their own expense. But even here the
picture is not so bleak since, as shown in table 15, the decline in tax
burdens in high-benefit states would free considerable state resources,
which could be used for such benefits. To avoid creating financial
difficulties for the most affected states during transition to a declining
matching-rate plan, a temporary limit could be placed on the amount
by which federal payments to any state would be allowed to change
in any year. It might be decided, for example, that irrespective of the
matching formula, federal payments (adjusted for inflation) could not
differ by more than 5 percent from the prior year's payments. This
way a state for which federal payments would ultimately fall (or rise)
by 30 percent would have the effect spread over about six years. While
states adversely affected would undoubtedly find reasons to object to
this plan, they cannot dispute the logic for the greater equity such a
system would provide.

Overall a declining-matching-rate formula with mandatory lump-
sum state contributions (designed to account for interstate differences
in medical care prices, taxpayers' income, and the number of poor
people) could be a useful means for moving toward the equity goals
we have set and would leave states with much freedom to develop
and administer their own Medicaid programs in ways that best meet
local needs.

Summary of Financing Alternatives

Before turning to a discussion of specific ways of controlling Medicaid
expenditures by shifting more responsibility to providers and recipients, we conclude our analysis of possible reforms of federal-state

TABLE 16
Overview of Simulated Financing Plans

Plan	Lowest as Percentage of Highest Benefit	Lowest as Percentage of Highest Tax Burden	State Cost as Percentage of Initial Cost	Federal Cost as Percentage of Initial Cost	Total Cost as Percentage of Initial Cost
Current matching[a]	16	11	100	100	100
Block grant at current level[a]	16	NA	0	100	55
4.5 percent reduction[a]	15	11	101	91	95
40 percent minimum matching[a]	16	11	100	94	97
Federalized at U.S. average	100	NA	0	182	100
Match to promote equal benefits[a]	100[b]	0[c,d]	84[d]	111[d]	99
Block grant with state contribution	100	100	100[d]	100[d]	100
Declining matching rate[a]	72	68[d]	99[d]	93[d]	96

NA = not applicable.
a. Simulation excludes Arizona.
b. Would actually be less than 100 percent because of random variations.
c. Reflects 100 percent matching for two states.
d. State and federal costs could be altered with a lump sum to achieve desired shares of costs and more nearly equal state tax burdens.

financing with a summary of the effects of various plans on recipient equity, taxpayer equity, and budgets. As a measure of recipient equity, the first column in table 16 shows, for each hypothetical plan, the benefits per poor person in the lowest-benefit state as a percentage of the comparable figure for the highest-benefit state. A perfectly equal distribution of benefits among the poor would produce a value of 100 in this column. This occurs only with the federalized plan and the block grant with state contribution, although the matching-rate schedule designed to produce equal benefits would come close. The particular version of the declining-matching-rate plan that we simulated also performed well for recipient equity, being much better on this count than the current system and better also than other moderate changes in matching that have been proposed in Congress.

As a measure of taxpayer equity, the second column shows the lowest state tax burden as a percentage of the highest state tax burden. Complete taxpayer equity is achieved only with the block grant with state contribution and (trivially) with federalization. The remaining columns show state, federal, and total costs, respectively, as a percentage of current costs. The figures are values for the particular simulations discussed above, but plans could be designed with similar structures to achieve more cost savings or to allow for greater benefits.

It appears that the last two plans discussed—block grants with state contributions and declining matching rates based on state demand—offer the best hope of producing a program that will measure up to the criteria of equity and demand satisfaction that we have chosen as our yardsticks. Neither of these plans resembles very closely any of the proposals for Medicaid cost control or "federalism" that have been discussed recently by Congress, the White House, or the National Governors' Association. Policy discussions in this area have included all-encompassing plans to federalize Medicaid—or large parts of Medicaid—and plans to chip away at Medicaid costs by reducing federal matching payments to states by small amounts. We have shown with the simulation results presented in this chapter that small changes in matching rates do not alter the basic inequities inherent in the program's current form. Moreover, the plans for uniform percentage-point reductions in matching rates that have received much attention could actually aggravate Medicaid's equity problems.

There is little more we can say about proposals to fully federalize Medicaid other than to point out that federalization must, it seems, eventually lead to uniform benefits among the states. Would benefits be set at a national average? The massive redistribution of Medicaid spending from the Northeast to other regions that this would entail may well not be politically acceptable. There would probably be pressure to increase total Medicaid spending to maintain benefit levels in the Northeast. While some redistribution is certainly desirable, identical benefit packages in every state may not be. A convincing rationale for full federalization has not yet been developed. If the purpose of federalization is to save costs, we can say with reasonable certainty that that is not a likely outcome, noting that the states have controlled the cost of Medicaid more effectively than the federal government has controlled the cost of Medicare. If the purpose is to promote equity among recipients and taxpayers, we can show how other means can be used to attain those objectives. If federalization is intended to provide fiscal relief to the states, we can remind ourselves that the burden is likely to be as great on the federal government. It is not necessary to discard the federal-state status of the Medicaid program to move toward the goals we have specified. We argue that the best course for Medicaid is in the direction of traditional federalism rather than federalization.

The most critical policy prescription seems to be as follows: since some states have higher benefits than others, some adjustment in federal-state financing relationships can help to bring about greater equity in the treatment of beneficiaries. With a simple matching-rate formula, such as the current one, taxpayer equity and beneficiary equity may eventually be in conflict as we try to reach our goals. The reason is that, although benefits are somewhat responsive to the price to users, getting benefits up to a national standard may, in some states, require a matching rate near 100 percent and consequently very low state Medicaid taxes. The inability to control both benefits and tax burdens with a single matching rate for each state can be overcome by combining matching rates with an appropriate block grant or lump-sum transfer between the federal government and each state.

A final consideration is that, although we can manipulate financial incentives to produce desired results, we still need to determine the national objectives concerning the level of Medicaid benefits. Recipient and taxpayer equity can be achieved at many different benefit levels, and federal incentives can be designed to make any of those levels state voting equilibriums. But which one is going to be a federal voting equilibrium? Is the level of benefits desired nationwide the high level in New York and Wisconsin, the low level in some southern states, or something in between?

There is, of course, no easy way to answer this. Although our empirical work does indicate the demand for the median voter in each state, it is difficult to know voters' demand for care for the poor outside their state. That is, although we can predict state responses to federal matching and can design plans to promote recipient and taxpayer equity, the optimal federal subsidy is harder to determine. Ultimately, the decision on benefits and eligibility must be a political one made at the federal level. It depends on taxpayers' attitudes toward poor people's consumption of medical care and, as eligibility is expanded, their willingness to subsidize those who are capable of contributing at least something toward the cost of their care. This problem must be resolved by the political process.

Notes

1. The computer simulations reported in this chapter are based on data for 1980, and the base line represents the situation before the 1981 Budget Reconciliation Act.

2. In economic terminology, a block grant has no price effect. There will be an income effect, but it is likely to be very small since Medicaid accounts for such a small share of the typical (median) voter's income. Some observers who have proposed bureaucratic or "flypaper" theories of governmental decision making believe that the income effect may be more important because a grant can be large in relation to a state government's budget. The authors of this study are skeptical of such theories except for short-run predictions. Such theories place the preferences of bureaucrats ahead of the preferences of voters, and this seems to be inconsistent with the practice of representative democracy, at least in the long run. A recent study of state and local AFDC expenditures found no evidence of the so-called flypaper effect when proper econometric techniques are applied. See Robert A. Moffitt, "The Effects of Grants-in-Aid on State and Local Expenditures: The Case of AFDC," paper presented at NBER Conference on Incentive Effects of Government Spending, Cambridge, Mass., November 1982.

3. Of course, states might be required to maintain some level of spending or otherwise contribute to program costs. We deal with mandatory state contributions below.

4. By optimal level of benefits we mean, as discussed above, the level at which the sum of in-state and out-of-state demand by voters is equal to the marginal cost of providing services.

5. The term "real Medicaid benefits" refers to dollar payments deflated by an index of the cost of medical care.

6. We use a price index that is a weighted average of hospital costs per patient-day, an index of physicians' fees, and local wage rates. Index values for each state are reported in appendix C.

7. C is the local cost of a standardized unit of medical care.

8. This is demonstrated in appendix A.

9. These include taxpayers' income, number of poor, local medical care prices, state racial composition, percentages of poor persons who are elderly or children, and regional effects. See Thomas Grannemann, "Reforming National Health Programs for the Poor," in Mark Pauly, ed., *National Health Insurance: What Now? What Later? What Never?* (Washington, D.C.: American Enterprise Institute, 1980).

10. The derivation of the formula to determine the state contribution is given in appendix A.

11. This provision could be modified to include some federal matching at the margin to assist states that wish to expand benefits beyond the standard level. This would mean, of course, relaxing our equity criteria to satisfy state preferences better and deal more appropriately with cross-state externalities.

12. Algebraically, the marginal matching rate for a given state is defined (over the relevant range 0 to 1) as

$$f = 1 - \frac{M - M_1^*}{M_2^* - M_1^*}$$

where f is the federal share at the margin and M is the state's medical vendor payments deflated by an index of state medical care prices. The variables M_1^* and M_2^* are defined as

$$M_1^* = 0.8 \times \bar{B}_{US} \times I \times N$$
$$M_2^* = 1.2 \times \bar{B}_{US} \times I \times N$$

where $\bar{B}_{US}$ is the average Medicaid payment per poor person in the United States, I is the state's index of medical care prices (I for the United States is 1.0), and N is the number of persons in the state below the poverty level.

13. Because U.S. poverty standards are not adjusted for local cost of living (except crudely for urban-rural differences), these rates are not fully adjusted for the real income of the poor. As a practical matter, however, this may not be a serious problem. The medical care price index (based on hospital cost per patient-day) results in higher matching rates where hospital costs are higher. This is appropriate, but we wish to avoid providing an incentive to raise the cost per day. This index partly reflects higher costs where hospital stays tend to be shorter and more service intensive (and more costly per day) rather than true differences in costs of producing care. Thus the medical care price index may overadjust for price differences, and the measure of number of poor underadjusts for cost-of-living differences. Because these two indexes are correlated, the two biases in our matching formula produce effects that tend to cancel each other. Nevertheless, a measure of poverty status that was fully adjusted for cost-of-living differences and a price index that was based on hospital (and nursing home) input prices rather than costs would make the matching rates more equitable.

14. Without such a contribution, state spending would be very small because the matching formula requires that the federal government pay the full cost up to the minimum level.

15. The lump-sum payment was calculated as

$$L = Y \times t - 0.125 \times (M_2^* - M_1^*)$$

where Y is aggregate adjusted gross income from individual tax returns; t is the average state tax burden (state share of Medicaid payments as fraction of taxpayer income) $= 0.006556$; M_2^* and M_1^* are as defined in note 12.

6
More Policy Options:
Direct Methods to Reduce
Medicaid Costs

An important question is whether there are ways of adjusting the benefit package offered to Medicaid beneficiaries so as to reduce the cost of care rendered to them in a way that minimizes the damage to the well-being of beneficiaries and taxpayers. There are two kinds of strategies that might be pursued to this end, either by the federal government or by states. The one that has been most frequently used and is most seriously discussed involves unilateral action by a single government-run insurance plan. Whatever action to reduce costs is undertaken—be it reduction in reimbursement rates, copayments, or whatever—all beneficiaries must accept the consequences that flow from a bureaucratic decision. A second approach relies on a sort of double-incentive structure to beneficiaries. One set of incentives is designed into a menu of insurance plans, some public but some privately offered, that encourage both beneficiaries and providers to reduce total expenditures. Another set of incentives guides the choice among plans by offering a greater reward for selecting a less costly plan. Beneficiaries could choose the plan that reduces costs in the way they most prefer; such an arrangement would also preserve freedom of choice, among providers and among plans, but modify that choice so that beneficiaries were rewarded for choosing plans that were less costly to taxpayers. While we favor the second approach, the methods for reducing costs discussed in this chapter could be pursued using either the unilateral-action or the incentive strategy.

Perhaps the best context in which to view the discussion of options for controlling cost is as advice to the states. In our view, the state should receive both the responsibility and the power to control costs; there is little virtue and may be some serious problems if a uniform set of policies is forced, from the federal level, on states with quite different taxpayer preferences, medical care delivery systems, and financial situations. It is not as if federal bureaucrats, or anyone else, really had a clear view of what pattern of medical care financing and medical care use is best for the poor; neither officials of the Department of Health and Human Services nor anyone else really knows what "works" when it comes to improving health, and there is even less knowledge about what improves general well-being —dignity, comfort, and so on.

It seems, therefore, a symptom of excessive pride for federal officials to write down restrictive regulations for the states. Instead, federal regulations should be permissive, reflecting the inchoate sentiments we all have that some more medical care in a general sense is desirable for the poor, but passing the question of exactly what care back down to the states. It also seems sensible for the states to pass the task of deciding how to spend a given sum further down, perhaps to local governments but, most important, to beneficiaries and their physician-advisers. There is, for example, no need that the same financing options, or the same set of rules, much less the same set of dollar standards, be applied to the inner-city areas of Chicago as to the very different rural areas in Illinois. Even within a given geographic area, different beneficiaries may sensibly choose different medical care plans.

Controlling Reimbursement Rates

Most of the policy discussion concerning reimbursement rates has dealt with possible limits on payments to providers, with a continuation of the Medicaid rule that prohibits supplementary payments from beneficiaries to providers. This basic strategy for limiting payments has been used for some time for physicians and other professionals. For institutions (hospitals and nursing homes), we have more limited experience with this approach in the somewhat different form of prospective payments—that is, payments based on rates set in advance and not dependent on costs incurred.

Payments to Physicians and Other Professionals. State Medicaid programs have been given considerable flexibility to determine how much will be paid for physicians' services. This flexibility has been used to lower payments, so that the average Medicaid payment for a visit to a physician is estimated to be only 65 percent of the average charge for visits of other patients. (Medicare pays about 84 percent on average.) Two empirically well documented facts are worthy of note. First, many physicians will not accept Medicaid patients or at least limit the number of their Medicaid patients, and the willingness to accept such patients varies predictably with the level of Medicaid payments.[1] Second, even though they are paid considerably less than the market price, many physicians are still willing to render services at Medicaid rates.

The first fact gives us a clue to what will happen if we attempt to control Medicaid costs by cutting physicians' fees further. We will further reduce access for the poor, in the sense that fewer physicians will be willing to accept Medicaid patients. We should be careful, however, about inferring from this that use of physicians' services will fall, much less that health will be affected. Although we have strong empirical documentation of the effect of the level of Medicaid payments to physicians on the willingness of physicians to accept Medicaid patients, we have very little information about the effect of this decision on the use of care. It may well be that the major effect of lower Medicaid payments is to reduce the set of physicians among whom the Medicaid patient can choose. In this sense, the debate about preserving free choice of providers in Medicaid is somewhat beside the point, at least when it comes to physicians' services; free choice has already been seriously abrogated. It may also be that the main effect of reduced access is primarily to impose implicit costs on beneficiaries; they are compelled to travel farther,[2] to use physicians with less convenient locations or hours, or to use types of providers (such as hospital outpatient departments or foreign medical school graduates) that they may not prefer.

The second fact indicates, however, that Medicaid payments to professionals can be reduced without causing the program to collapse; costs can be cut, at least costs per unit. Do we know the effect on total costs for physicians' services? It may be that physicians respond to lower prices by delivering less quality and more quantity, especially since it is nearly impossible for the government to monitor what is actually being provided. If the payment per visit is cut, for example, the physician may choose to treat a case with two ten-minute visits rather than one twenty-minute visit, even though both the physician and the patient might much prefer the single longer visit.

Trying to save money by limiting payment to physicians for their services may not be the best way to use the structure of payments to physicians to reduce program costs. Total payments to physicians for their services constitute a relatively small fraction of total Medicaid costs—8 percent in fiscal 1980. But many other services are highly complementary to physicians' services, and the physician controls the use of those services to a great degree. By restructuring fee schedules or encouraging prepaid group practices so that we reward the physician for lower hospital, nursing home, laboratory, or prescription drug costs, we may actually save more even if physicians are paid more. This is a delicate matter, of course. Paying the physician more for surgery if it is conducted in a less costly outpatient setting may cause the physician to switch the place at which surgery is performed, but it may also bring about more surgery.

Payments to Hospitals. In contrast to the arrangements for physicians' services, Medicaid has generally been required to pay hospitals on the same basis as Medicare. Through most of the course of both programs, this has meant payment of the program's share of whatever each hospital's cost happened to be, with arguments limited to the appropriate share of the two government programs in the total cost. With the passage of the 1972 amendments to the Social Security Act, however, there has begun a gradual but consistent trend toward paying less than actual cost to unusually high cost hospitals under provision of section 223 of that law.[3] Section 223 limits have probably reduced the revenue paid by the government to some hospitals, although they have yet to have a major impact. It is not clear what effect they have had on the cost of providing care. Section 223 limits may also have resulted in the transfer of costs for public patients to other patients and their insurance companies.

Many states have adopted some form of hospital rate review or prospective reimbursement system. In some states rate setting applies only to Medicaid, and in others the rates apply to all payers. The evidence on the effect of rate review is somewhat ambiguous, but it does suggest on balance that rate review has reduced both hospital revenue per unit and total revenue in those states in which it has been implemented. What is uncertain is the effect of these programs on cost. There is some evidence that in the early years of the New York state revenue limits, hospitals responded not by cutting costs but by running deficits and eating up their capital. Econometric estimates by Sloan and Steinwald of the effect of prospective reimbursement on hospital costs through 1975 were small.[4] But there is evidence that in later years prospective rate-setting programs have been associated with lower rates of growth in costs.[5]

A form of prospective reimbursement that has recently received much attention is payment by diagnostic related groups (DRGs). In a DRG system hospitals receive a single fixed payment for each admission based on the patient's diagnosis. Such a plan has been implemented statewide in New Jersey for all payers, public and private, and in early 1983 a DRG system for Medicare was hastily adopted by Congress. Compared with other prospective rate plans, DRG schemes pay a fixed amount per hospital stay rather than per day or per service. This provides hospitals with incentives to reduce use of ancillary services and to keep hospital stays as short as possible.

DRG systems provide no direct incentives, however, for physicians or patients to limit use of services during a stay and, in fact, eliminate such incentives for those patients who pay for at least part of the cost of their care. The effectiveness of a DRG system, therefore, depends on the ability of hospital administrators to alter the behavior of physicians in ordering services and discharging patients. DRG-based reimbursement also sets up incentives for hospitals to encourage multiple admissions to treat a single illness and admission of less severely ill patients with low expected service needs relative to others in a diagnostic category, and to discourage admission of severely ill patients. Hospitals reimbursed by DRGs would probably attempt to attract patients in categories for which reimbursement is relatively generous and might find creative ways to assign (perhaps even through misrepresentation) patients to the highest-cost DRG category possible. It is still too early to tell from the New Jersey experience how important these incentives will be and in the end what effect DRGs will have on use of services, quality of care, and costs.

If the amount Medicaid and Medicare will pay to hospitals is further reduced through any type of prospective payment system, several responses can be anticipated. First, access is likely to be reduced. If they are permitted to do so, some hospitals may refuse public patients altogether. Others may try in more subtle ways to curb provision of services to public patients—by limiting outreach programs, by judicious transfers to other hospitals, by enlisting the aid of their physician staff. In addition, some reduction in quality or intensity of care is likely. Here again we do not know the form it will take: Will clinical quality be cut, will amenities be reduced, or what? Relative reductions in quality or amenities are most likely to occur in those hospital departments that are heavily patronized by Medicaid patients, such as the ambulatory care departments.

What of inefficiency, or "fat"? Probably some will be cut, although we do not know how much, mostly because we do not know how much there is. But it is virtually certain that not all of the adjustment will come out of technical and input price inefficiency; there is no way to target only inefficiency. There will have to be some reduction in the real quality of care rendered to Medicaid beneficiaries.

Medicaid beneficiaries tend to be heavy users of hospital outpatient facilities, and the unit price for those services tends to be higher than for similar services rendered in a physician's office. Where hospitals are reimbursed the lesser of costs or charges for providing outpatient care but face limits on the inpatient side, price differences may be the result of a hospital pricing policy that tries to make profit on outpatient facilities by ensuring that as many costs as possible are allocated to the outpatient unit and that charges always exceed those accounting measures of costs. The unknown here is whether the economic marginal cost of hospital-provided outpatient care differs from that of similar care provided by physicians in private practice. It does seem obvious that a reduction in what Medicaid pays for outpatient care will tend to reduce access for beneficiaries and possibly to reduce quality as well. Hospitals have typically not refused Medicaid patients, partly because as long as Medicaid paid like Medicare and both paid cost there was no need to refuse service and partly because past receipt of Hill-Burton funds was interpreted as committing the hospital to provide some free care. If Medicaid cuts back on hospital reimbursement, however, it is only fair to permit hospitals with costs greater than reimbursement to refuse to provide nonemergency services or to provide services to Medicaid beneficiaries at a lower level of style or amenity. One reason is that the willingness of Medicaid to pay costs implied a kind of social contract between taxpayers and hospitals to pay for the kind of care hospitals were providing. If the taxpayers abrogate their part of this contract by reducing reimbursement, it would not be equitable to expect hospitals to uphold their part and continue providing high-cost care at the expense of other users or their employees.

If hospitals are required to provide service when revenue is less than cost, they will have to cover the loss somehow. If they consume working capital, they will eventually cease to be able to provide service to anyone. Trying to charge other patients more may not be feasible in a competitive system; even if it is, financing care for the poor with what amounts to an excise tax levied on hospital care for the nonpoor is both inefficient and, in a sense, politically dishonest. Covering losses with additional voluntary community donations is perhaps the least damaging method, but the required scale makes it infeasible in many areas, and in any case it suffers from the inequity of having local charity support a program of state and national benefit. Finally, requiring hospitals to continue to render service really defeats the social purpose of cost cutting. The object, after all, is to reduce the amount of resources flowing into medical care. If some hospital care is judged to be too costly in relation to its benefits, the proper action is to ensure that the care is not provided, whether it be the expensive outpatient visit for a minor illness or an unnecessarily long inpatient hospital stay. Cutting what the government pays but requiring services to be provided does not cut the real resource costs—the same resources will have to be used to produce the same care. It does affect how services are financed, shifting the costs from government budgets to higher charges for hospital care to nonpoor patients. However better off this may make government administrators and however much it cuts taxes, it does not really improve and may even worsen taxpayers' overall well-being.

One additional aspect of reducing payments to hospitals and physicians should be discussed. As the payer for both Medicaid and Medicare services, the federal government has considerable buying power in the medical care market—not as much as if it controlled the entire market, but still some. This gives the federal government some monopsony power—the power to influence the prices it pays for services—which it may be able and willing to use to keep hospital and physician costs down for Medicare and Medicaid. The use of monopsony power is normally thought to lead to economic inefficiency, which in this case means the government might, in attempting to reduce costs, set payments so low that too little care would be provided. It is quite difficult to judge the economic efficiency of such arrangements, however, since the reduction in use that would result might simply offset the incentive insurance provides for overuse.

If payments to providers should be further reduced, one possible improvement in Medicaid policy would be to permit beneficiaries to supplement Medicaid payments with payments of their own. The beneficiary who must travel for care because a close-by physician is unwilling to accept Medicaid may gain by being permitted to make up the difference between the Medicaid payment and the doctor's going price. Presumably, the restriction on supplementation by beneficiaries is intended to prevent beneficiaries from being "ripped off"; yet an arrangement that permits supplementation seems to work reasonably well for Medicare. Permitting supplementation may reduce government monopsony power, but a beneficiary faced with the choice of no care at a zero out-of-pocket price or care that he or she likes with a small positive supplementation may prefer the latter.

Contractual and Prudent Buyer Arrangements

A fundamental premise we have emphasized throughout this study is that any reductions in Medicaid spending should be made in a way that minimizes damage to the overall welfare of Medicaid recipients. If the government wants to reduce public outlays, what features of the program seem likely to yield the least painful cuts? Some have suggested that access—as embodied in the "freedom of choice" provision of Medicaid—is one such feature. With some exceptions permitted by the 1981 Budget Reconciliation Act, Medicaid beneficiaries can now select whichever provider they wish from all those providers willing to serve them. But how can we restrict Medicaid beneficiaries to use of low-cost providers without severely impairing their access to care?

From an economic viewpoint, recent debate over removing or retaining free choice has missed an important point. Freedom of choice is excess baggage once a reimbursement level is set. For a transaction to take place in any market, the customer must be willing to buy, and the seller must be willing to sell. If the price that will be paid to the seller is too low, the transaction will not occur, even if the patient desires to use the provider's services. The zero user price for Medicaid usually eliminates the willingness of the buyer as a binding constraint. If the state does not want a particular transaction to occur, it can prevent it by setting what the supplier receives below the supplier's minimum price; there is no need to restrict freedom of choice of buyers directly. Setting a price high enough to bring forth extra supply but then limiting freedom of choice so as to exclude some providers is an inferior strategy; the need to limit freedom of choice means that the price is set higher than is necessary to induce supply of the desired quantity of services.

These comments serve to point out that the response by physicians to low reimbursement levels—that is, refusing to participate in Medicaid—already seriously circumscribes freedom of choice. If, in the future, hospitals are also able and willing to respond to reductions in real payments to them by withholding services, freedom will be further restricted. In short, actual (or economic) freedom of choice is probably already much more restrictive than possible regulatory approaches to limiting free choice of providers.

The critical point, however, is that supply responses to lower reimbursement rates can be an efficient and effective means of cutting costs; but then regulatory limits on demand or freedom of choice are unnecessary and clearly inferior. It may be possible and preferable to cut costs while keeping present levels of regulatory freedom of choice for Medicaid beneficiaries. The reason for preserving the beneficiaries' freedom to choose is that, within the limits imposed by licensure and participation standards, patients are presumably better off if they are allowed to choose the provider who pleases them most, if that provider is willing to accept what is paid on their behalf. What is to be paid by public insurance reflects taxpayers' judgment about the value of care to the poor. If poor people can select care that they prefer and that carries a cost not exceeding what taxpayers are willing to pay, no one is better off by further restricting choice; there is no gain from restriction. More important, free choice can be expanded, at no cost to the taxpayers, by fixing the level of Medicaid payments and permitting beneficiaries to supplement the amounts Medicaid pays to providers.

This is not to imply that such free choice will not be objectionable to some. For the process to work in the way described, suppliers must be permitted to refuse to serve. Thus there is a casualty of cost cutting: the ideal of "no two-class medicine" will have to be sacrificed. In fact, of course, the reality never corresponded to the ideal; some physicians always refused Medicaid patients for whom they were poorly reimbursed, and access for beneficiaries was low because costs to providers for treating them were high in relation to the revenues received. More important, however, a single-class premium-quality medicine is an ideal that is probably neither affordable nor—when alternatives are considered—preferable. Taxpayers, it appears, are not willing to pay the cost of this objective. An acceptable level of care for the poor, at an acceptable cost, is probably a more reasonable goal. Unless one attaches a very strong value to equity, any single amenity standard is probably not optimal.

As a practical matter, however, one can ask whether a program with freedom of choice can be as cheap as prudent buyer plans (such as those being tried by some states under the waiver regulations of the 1981 Budget Reconciliation Act) that restrict beneficiaries to the use of providers who meet state cost, quality, and use requirements. The answer is that it can, if the Medicaid reimbursement for any beneficiary is limited to what would have been paid to those providers from whom the state would have purchased services. The new Arizona Medicaid program, for example, has put out various types of care for per capita bids, the counties themselves (which have heretofore provided care to the indigent in Arizona) as well as private sector providers competing for prepaid contracts. The most obvious way to preserve freedom of choice is to have bids and give a voucher equal in value to the lowest bid to any Medicaid beneficiary who does not want to use the "winning" system. Medicaid beneficiaries could supplement that voucher if they wished to purchase more costly care elsewhere, and they could share in the savings if they found an even cheaper source than the county or institution that was the low bidder.

In general, where the mechanisms are in place, it seems appropriate that county or municipal public hospitals should serve as a backbone of a free choice system. They could be the "suppliers of first resort," the choice of care for a beneficiary with indifferent preferences. But if more attractive care—however the beneficiary judges attractiveness—can be obtained elsewhere at the same cost to taxpayers, there seems to be no reason to require that Medicaid beneficiaries use a publicly operated system or be prohibited from using the provider of their choice if they are willing to pay the extra cost. Although allowing beneficiaries to supplement Medicaid reimbursement may erode the government's monopsony power to some extent, it should broaden the range of providers who compete to serve Medicaid patients. With improved access for Medicaid recipients, the government may even be willing to set reimbursement rates lower than otherwise, and if supplementation became the norm, it would give recipients incentives to limit their use of services of low value.

Is it plausible to think that poor people would or should have supplementable vouchers? First, we know that poor people who are not eligible for Medicaid do spend money out of pocket on medical care, so that it is not true that the poor cannot "afford" to pay something for more attractive or convenient care. We even have some direct evidence that medically needy Medicaid beneficiaries are willing and able to share in the cost of prepayment plan premiums and that they are also willing to pay higher premiums to maintain an existing relationship with a family doctor.[6] Second, some providers may have marginal costs below the average and may be willing to accept a lower payment for some of their patients. Indeed, the voucher arrangement is the logical implementation of competitive principles, whereas the prudent buyer concept is inimical to competition and may only serve to shield established but inefficient publicly operated institutions from competition. A multiple-choice strategy will not be especially effective in rural areas where there are few providers, but even there it will do little harm.

Health Maintenance Organizations

The health maintenance organization (HMO), or prepaid group practice, has been much discussed as a method of controlling medical care costs, and for that reason we need not get into a detailed discussion of HMOs. The evidence available is that those enrolled in HMOs tend to have lower costs, mainly because of lower rates of hospitalization. It is not clear, however, how much of the reduced use is attributable to what the HMO does and how much is due to self-selection of the HMO by low users.[7] In any case, the cost experience of HMOs may not fairly represent the cost-saving potential of using HMOs in various ways under Medicaid. Much of the evidence on HMO costs is based on comparisons within groups of union members and government employees. To attract members from these relatively high income groups, the HMOs may have offered more high-quality features and amenities than might be considered essential by lower-income individuals and families. Until recently even Medicaid recipients have had no reason to choose an HMO if it did not offer features and amenities that they valued more highly than the option of unlimited care at no out-of-pocket cost in the fee-for-service sector. Now, however, with the passage of the 1981 Budget Reconciliation Act, states may, under waiver, enroll Medicaid recipients in an accessible HMO and restrict their use of other providers. It remains to be seen how states will make use of this provision and whether costs will be reduced as a result.

Under an HMO arrangement beneficiaries do lose something. At a minimum, they lose freedom to change providers at will, and they may also lose access to the most convenient or most preferred provider, perhaps one with whom they have an existing relationship. And they may lose the extra medical care that would have been supplied by fee-for-service providers. This might be viewed as a meaningful loss, at least by some people with some sets of preferences, but others might consider such services unnecessary. Of course, membership in an HMO is usually voluntary; so we see few examples of persons actually made worse off by joining an HMO. Nevertheless, the potential for underproviding care is clearly present in the HMO concept unless competition is very strong. For this reason HMO enrollment for Medicaid recipients would probably work best in connection with some form of voucher plan so that the recipients could change plans if they were dissatisfied with the services provided. In any case, competition for the private-pay members should keep the HMO services at an acceptable level if there are alternative sources of care in the local area and if Medicaid recipients without other reasonable options do not constitute too large a share of the HMOs' membership.[8]

Copayments

Another device to reduce use by bringing about a comparison of costs and benefits is to require payments by users. Copayments force the beneficiary to ask whether the care is really worth paying something for and therefore constitute an ideal mechanism for eliminating services not highly valued by Medicaid recipients themselves. As with any medical insurance plan, there is a trade-off to be made between reducing exposure to financial risk and improving incentives to consider the cost of care—that is, minimizing the moral hazard problem. We may be more worried about the financial risk of high medical expenses for low-income persons than for other groups. But there is certainly room to introduce moderate copayments for routine primary care services, and small percentage copayments for hospital services might be tolerable as well, provided an upper annual limit was placed on a recipient family's copayments.

Early results from the Health Insurance Study, in which families were randomly assigned to insurance plans with various copayment schemes, confirm economic logic by showing that copayments do in fact reduce expenditures on medical services. Perhaps somewhat more important for Medicaid is the preliminary finding that the effect of copayments—at least with income-related upper limits—did not vary significantly with the participating family's income.[9] Fears that even small copayments would result in drastic reductions in use by the poor appear to be unfounded. For purposes of Medicaid, the ideal copayment plan would set an upper limit on total payments and might well employ a multiple-choice voucher arrangement. This would allow the beneficiaries themselves to choose the degree of risk they wish to assume and permit them to share in savings from plans with higher copayments.

Reforming Long-Term Care

Unlike virtually all other insurance plans—public or private—Medicaid covers long-term nursing home care. Medicaid's coverage of nursing home care, with no comparable coverage of home care, has created an incentive for some elderly recipients and their families to choose nursing home placement rather than attempt to deal with the problems and costs of living in the community. It has been widely recognized that, for some elderly persons, home care may offer a preferred and possibly less expensive alternative to institutional care. One common suggestion, therefore, is to extend Medicaid coverage to services that would permit an impaired elderly person in need of assistance to remain outside an institution. It is evident, however, that even those elderly persons not likely to enter a nursing home have a large capacity for making use of community-based services such as home health aides, homemakers, and home-delivered meals, especially when they are free. Any uncontrolled expansion of home care benefits is likely to increase the cost of serving this "not-at-risk" group by more than it reduces costs for potential nursing home residents. If we are looking for ways to save Medicaid costs, a means must be found to limit public funding of home services to situations in which it is most likely to reduce institutional care.

A mechanism that has received much attention in the literature is public coordination of formal community-based services and informal (largely family) supports, but the cost-saving effects of this case management approach have not yet been proved. States have been given permission to experiment with this approach under waivers authorized by section 2176 of the 1981 Budget Reconciliation Act, but the most definitive evidence on the effects of case management should come from the National Long Term Care Channeling Demonstration. In the demonstration, local "channeling" projects attempt to identify elderly clients at risk of entering a nursing home, conduct individual needs assessment and care planning, and coordinate delivery of community-based services. At some of the sites, channeling projects directly contract with providers for delivery of services, giving the projects some degree of local monopsony power that could lower prices or improve service. The success of these projects in reducing Medicaid costs and meeting other objectives will not be known, however, until the demonstration is completed in 1985. One disadvantage of the case management approach is that it reduces clients' ability to choose their own providers. This, however, might be viewed as a small price to pay for opening up the option for some elderly persons to remain at home in the community rather than enter a nursing home.

Most recent discussion of long-term-care policy has focused on ways of meeting the immediate needs of the elderly. Less attention has been devoted to investigating the possibility of dealing with the risks to low-income elderly persons over a longer time. Many elderly Medicaid recipients are low-income persons whose resources have been depleted because of expenses incurred during unanticipated prolonged periods of poor health or simply the unplanned-for expenses of living longer than expected. Such low-income persons may really need only some form of affordable long-term-care insurance to cover such risks. Although the current Medicaid system offers some limited protection, elderly persons are often forced to spend down into poverty to become eligible for Medicaid. There are ways of avoiding this situation and of decentralizing decisions on eligibility and the determination of need by permitting the option of contracting out long-term-care insurance in an HMO-like fashion.

A number of practical problems would need to be overcome in such a plan. First, there is the problem of adverse selection (that is, only the relatively unhealthy sign up). To avoid adverse selection, the enrollment decision could be required well before the need for long-term care arises. For example, low-income persons in reasonably good health could be told at age sixty-five that they are entitled to a certain dollar amount of nursing home and home care insurance benefits under Medicaid—as long as they also make a commitment at age sixty-five to which "plan" they will use. Their benefits would then be assigned to that plan up to the full amount of the plan's premium. Qualifying plans would be required to demonstrate the financial and operational capability of providing care but could charge more or less than the standard premium. In this way, the consumer could choose the strictness of the eligibility criteria and the amount of premium he or she is to pay. Under this approach, a plan could pay for care at home, even to family members, or could require use of the least costly form of care for the beneficiary. Savings would be provided to the individual in the form of a lower premium. The government could make premium payments to private plans for persons deemed incapable of paying, and persons who through inheritance or other means were no longer needy could have their government premium subsidy terminated.

A second potential problem is that the plans may not in practice be able to implement cost control in a superior way, although there is every reason to assume they could do at least as well as public sector case management agencies.

A third problem is ensuring a plan's ability to pay benefits, because in agreeing to deliver services for a lump sum or level premium, the plan must forecast future nursing home and home health prices. One solution would be to raise the government's premium subsidy in proportion to some price index, the base being the premium in some base year. Another approach would be to permit plans to elect their own investment strategies, subject to minimal constraints on the amount of care provided, and allow the financial markets to deal with the problem of uncertainty over future prices.

A final possible problem relates to the minimal optimal scale of such plans. Since it is not clear just what functions suppliers of long-term-care insurance would perform, the technology is uncertain; but if plans are to monitor current needs for service of beneficiaries, some local presence would be required. If the number of beneficiaries in need of services in an area at any one time—and this would be a small fraction of those enrolled—were too small to operate a plan cost effectively, the long-term-care insurance plan would be a natural monopoly. That is, there might not be room for more than one plan of efficient size in the local market. In many areas there does appear to be room for more than one provider of home health aides and homemakers, however; so if the long-term-care insurance plans were integrated with service providers, the overhead costs of an office and administrative staff might be minimized, and trained clinical staff might be employed productively in other activities when not needed for work assessing the needs of beneficiaries.

Removing Ineligible Recipients from the Rolls

No study of Medicaid cost control would be complete without some mention of the benefits being provided to persons who are not legally entitled to them. Very little information is available on how many ineligible persons are receiving Medicaid benefits. If state administrators knew how to identify such persons at some reasonable cost, they would not be giving them benefits; and state administrators who do not know how to identify ineligible recipients understandably do not talk much about it. All we can say is that professionals who deal directly with low-income groups can often describe cases of persons getting Medicaid benefits illegally.

A typical situation is that of a two-parent family that would otherwise be eligible for Medicaid but is not eligible because the program excludes households where both parents are present. Some such families may deceitfully report the father or mother as continually absent from the household to qualify. Because continued absence is expensive for the state to monitor, the family can usually claim benefits without difficulty if it chooses, even if the second parent is generally present. Another situation that arises frequently is that a Medicaid recipient loses eligibility by going back to work after a period of unemployment. Since this is also difficult for the state to discover, benefits may continue for some time unless the recipient reports the change in employment status.

In a third situation assets above the limit for eligibility are concealed or transferred. Unlike the previous two examples, this problem may be more frequent among elderly recipients than AFDC families. Medicaid in effect imposes a 100 percent tax on assets by requiring individuals to deplete their own assets before obtaining Medicaid eligibility. This provides an incentive for elderly persons to transfer assets illegally to their families before entering a nursing home. These transactions go largely undetected and may even take place before the person applies for eligibility. Strict enforcement of the current eligibility requirements in any of these cases would be costly and would require some intrusion in the private affairs of recipients.

There are four possible strategies for policy in this area: allow the current situation to persist, vigorously prosecute a few cases and hope potential offenders will be deterred, incur the enforcement costs and tolerate some intrusion on recipients' privacy, or change the eligibility requirements so that they can be enforced. Perhaps the best approach under the circumstances would be some combination of these strategies. We could do away with some of the hard-to-enforce categorical eligibility requirements that benefit people who cheat at the expense of those who are honest. In addition, enforcement could be stepped up, and states could be encouraged to make use of various data bases to identify sources of income and assets of beneficiaries. Proper safeguards for privacy should be established, of course, but letting the state welfare office know how much we make so they can provide benefits to those of us who really need them seems no more of an evil than letting the Internal Revenue Service know our incomes so it can take money from those of us who have it.

Notes

1. Frank Sloan, Janet Mitchell, and Jerry Cromwell, "Physician Participation in State Medicaid Programs," *Journal of Human Resources*, vol. 13 (Supplement 1978), pp. 211–45; Philip J. Held, John Holahan, and Cathy Carlson, "The Effect of Medicaid and Private Fees on Physician Participation in California's Medicaid Program, 1974–1978," Urban Institute Working Paper 1306-02-04, March 1982.

2. Some direct evidence comes from a recent evaluation of the National Health Service Corps (NHSC) in rural areas, in which it was found that, among NHSC office visits, Medicaid patients took longer (and presumably traveled farther) to reach the physician's office than non-Medicaid patients. See Thomas Grannemann, Francesca Seidita, and Mark Pauly, *An Analysis of the Content of Office Visits Provided by NHSC and Private-Sector Physicians*, project report, Mathematica Policy Research, Inc., 1982.

3. Public law 92-603, section 223, excludes from the definition of reasonable cost "any part of incurred cost found to be unnecessary in the efficient delivery of needed health services." The open-endedness of this provision has led some to suggest it as a possible means of sharply reducing payments to hospitals without the need for further legislation.

4. Frank Sloan and Bruce Steinwald, *Insurance, Regulation, and Hospital Costs* (Lexington, Mass.: D. C. Heath, 1980).

5. See Craig Coelen and Daniel Sullivan, "An Analysis of the Effects of Prospective Reimbursement Programs on Hospital Expenditures," *Health Care Financing Review*, vol. 2, no. 3 (Winter 1981), pp. 1–40; and Brian Biles, Carl Schram, and J. Graham Atkinson, "Hospital Cost Inflation under State Rate-Setting Programs," *New England Journal of Medicine*, vol. 303, no. 12 (September 18, 1980).

6. Trudi W. Galblum and Sidney Trieger, "Demonstration of Alternative Delivery Systems under Medicare and Medicaid," *Health Care Financing Review*, vol. 3, no. 3 (March 1982), summarizing a report on Project Health by Jurgovan and Blair, Inc.

7. For a more complete discussion of the evidence on HMOs, see Harold S. Luft, *Health Maintenance Organizations* (New York: Wiley, 1981).

8. For a brief review of some of the problems of implementing HMO plans under Medicaid, see Galblum and Trieger, "Demonstration of Alternative Delivery Systems." Luft, *Health Maintenance Organizations,* chap. 13, also discusses using HMOs to serve the poor.

9. See Joseph Newhouse et al., "Some Interim Results from a Controlled Trial of Cost Sharing in Health Insurance," *New England Journal of Medicine,* vol. 305, no. 25 (December 17, 1981), pp. 1501–7.

7

Improving Medicaid and Controlling Cost

In this chapter we spell out our preferred set of policies in more detail. There is a group of reforms for Medicaid that can contribute to controlling cost in a way that minimizes harm to potential beneficiaries. The fundamental idea is that, rather than have decisions centralized at the federal level, it is preferable to decentralize as much as possible: some decisions to the states and many decisions to the Medicaid beneficiaries themselves.

The success of any form of the Medicaid program depends, to a considerable extent, on the amount of resources committed to the program. But the suggestions we make for improving the efficiency of the program are, we believe, desirable no matter what level of funding is chosen. The changes we suggest will give voters a better view of and better control over the kind of medical care they are buying for the poor, and voters may be inclined to devote more public dollars to a program that produces better results per dollar.

We consider two broad kinds of reform: The first deals with the way the beneficiary should relate to whatever level of government is administering the program. The second deals with the appropriate assignment of financing and control to the various levels of government. Both will help voters to exercise their generosity in the most appropriate way and to the most appropriate extent.

Beneficiary Choice Medicaid

In this section we propose an alternative way of reducing Medicaid cost that operates by using choice in the private market. Our basic objective is to preserve free choice and still give Medicaid beneficiaries incentives to be concerned about cost. Current reimbursement methods leave the beneficiary with little effective choice of primary care providers once the level of payments has been determined. Prudent buyer or contract-type arrangements would reduce choice still further. We will outline the essential elements of a program that, rather than compelling the beneficiary to use a less preferred provider who happens to be cheaper, gives beneficiaries incentives to develop low-cost patterns of care by sharing any savings with them. This approach, which we call beneficiary choice Medicaid, is a generalization of the voucher idea, but with fewer restrictions and more options than in most proposed voucher programs.

The idea is simple. A state government would define a standard set of Medicaid benefits. This set could most conveniently be thought of as similar to current benefits, but it could also be a different set depending on the state's preferences. For any household of given characteristics, this insurance package would have an actuarial value equal to the average expenditure per beneficiary unit of that type. A Medicaid household would be permitted to purchase health insurance and health care from alternative sources as long as certain minimum benefit standards were met. If the total cost of care under the alternative were less than the actuarial value (in an expected value or average sense), the household would be rewarded with some fraction of the cost savings. If the cost were more, the household would be permitted to enroll in the plan and pay the difference. Alternative packages that would deliver a little less (in freedom of choice, convenience, amenities, access, or quality) than the state's established standard benefit package but cost less would then be available to beneficiaries. In return for selecting a lower-cost package, beneficiaries would receive a reward proportional to the cost savings associated with each alternative. Health plans,[1] HMOs, and other such novel but so far uncommon health insurance arrangements would become feasible and attractive, at least to some Medicaid beneficiaries. Other cost-reducing arrangements, such as copayments, deductibles, per-unit indemnities, and per-case indemnities, which are available now, would also become possible features of plans available as options to Medicaid beneficiaries.

Whatever level of expenditure or expenditure reduction a state wanted to set, this approach would permit beneficiaries themselves, rather than bureaucrats, to decide what they were willing to do without. Some beneficiaries, of course, would decide to keep benefits at current levels, perhaps with some supplementation out of their own pockets. Most beneficiaries who find a lower-cost insurer would probably use some of the incentive payments to add different benefits to the standard package, although the program would permit them to take the savings in cash—to be used for better housing, more adequate diet, education, recreation, or whatever they prefer. In effect, this approach would be a small step toward "cashing out" Medicaid services of low marginal value to the recipient, a step that might at least moderate the need for increases in cash benefit programs. To ensure that all recipients would have access to basic services, some minimum level of benefits could be mandated for programs that qualify.

A variety of plan features would be likely to emerge under beneficiary choice Medicaid. A method that produces cost savings in principle is the closed-panel health plan, in either its HMO variant or some less formalized structure. A "cost-saving sharing percentage" (for example, 60 percent) could be established for any cost saving in relation to the standard plan's actuarial cost, adjusted for the recipient's age, sex, family status, and presence of chronic conditions. Suppose the actuarial value of the state's standard plan for a family were $3,000 but a particular health plan could deliver the same benefits for $2,500. A beneficiary could choose either the standard plan or the new plan and up to $300 ($500 × 0.60) worth of additional benefits.

Another option, and one easier to implement now, would be to identify a set of providers with low unit costs and give beneficiaries incentives to use those providers. An arrangement like the Newhouse-Taylor variable cost (per unit indemnity) insurance would be one form of this idea.[2] Suppose, for example, that a select set of hospitals in a metropolitan area can be found with costs per admission 20 percent below average. Beneficiaries who agree in advance to use those hospitals can be rewarded with 12 percent of the fraction of Medicaid payments that would have gone to hospitals. Should they in fact use more expensive hospitals, their prospective dividends can be applied to the additional cost.

For some procedures, specific indemnities per case would be possible, and here again there could be sharing of cost savings. For example, with a 60 percent cost-savings sharing percentage, obstetricians who agreed to provide normal deliveries for 20 percent less than average could generate a credit to their patients of 12 percent of the average amount.

What is missing in the present system is some way of capturing savings from the effects on use of various kinds of copayments, without at the same time cutting into Medicaid beneficiaries' real income or increasing cash outlays by the government. We cannot know for sure, until such a system of copayments and deductibles is tried, if it would be effective enough to achieve this combined objective, but we can consider some plausible numbers. Suppose a $100 hospital deductible reduced admissions by 10 percent. With a cost per admission of over $1,000, the savings would be large enough to return more money to beneficiaries, on the average, than they pay in deductibles. Of course, such a plan would benefit most those people who used less care and would leave beneficiaries with multiple hospitalizations with less money to spend on other things.

Beneficiary choice provisions would not necessarily alter Medicaid eligibility criteria. But with known costs of the participating health plans, it would be possible to allow low-income persons who are not currently eligible to buy into the plan of their choice, possibly at a publicly subsidized rate related to the person's income. The unemployed could have the premium deducted from their unemployment checks, and the deduction might even be made mandatory for those who were without other health insurance. Depending on the amount of subsidy, if any, serving these groups could raise Medicaid costs; but in the end taxpayers might not be worse off than they are at present as much of the cost of care for these individuals now shows up in bad debts to providers, budgets of public hospitals, and other state and local programs.

The precise form and parameters of state beneficiary choice programs would need to be determined by state legislatures, and the extent to which beneficiaries would make use of the options cannot be known now. Accordingly, it is not possible either to suggest an ideal program design or to estimate with any precision how much such a plan might save state and federal governments. The features of a sample beneficiary choice program are outlined in appendix B.

The Ideal Level of Government for Medicaid Functions

Like education, medical care is something whose quality and outcomes are perhaps best judged by those closest to the users of the service. Federal policy makers and administrators can only specify rules and regulations that must be applied in a wide variety of circumstances. They cannot be aware of the implications of their decisions for every case, or even for every class of cases. A rule that is too restrictive in one locality may work very well in a place where alternative public health programs are available to the poor. The difficulty of ensuring good performance of Medicaid from Washington is evident in the numerous instances reported in the press of deserving persons denied appropriate care. A prominent example is the case of Katie Becket, a disabled child who was not allowed to receive care at home under Medicaid. After her case came to the attention of President Reagan, Health and Human Services Secretary Richard Schweiker formed a board to review similar cases. One wonders, first, why it took the federal government so long to recognize this problem and, second, whether cabinet-level decision making is really required in such matters. For purposes of administering Medicaid—determining how a given amount of money should be spent, who should be eligible, and how costs should be controlled— our view is that states are better suited than the federal government.

The fundamental flaw in the argument for federalization is the implicit assumption that the federal government knows or can ever know what is the "right" thing to do. As we have noted, determining how to spend the money is not subject to precise evaluation, and so we are left with the traditional argument for retaining authority at lower levels of government: because they are closer to voters and program outcomes, lower levels of government are to be preferred unless there is a clear reason to the contrary. At most, there may be modest economies of scale in administration at a more centralized level, but even these can be captured by small states if they contract out those functions. In many states, for example, claims processing is already handled by firms that have contracts to provide similar services for other states.

The problem of financing is more complex. For the reason we discussed above, the ideal arrangement is one in which the financing responsibility is shared by the state and federal governments—the federal government operating not as an independent entity but as a representative of persons elsewhere in the country who are concerned about the health, the use of medical care, and the well-being of the poor nationwide. Ultimately, then, the financing mechanism should be one that both distributes costs equitably between taxpayers in the state and outside and leads voters in each state to choose a level of total expenditures that reflects the benevolence and sense of equity of voters inside and outside the state.

The federal government also has an important role in providing technical assistance to the states to avoid duplication of efforts. In developing the Medicaid Management Information System (MMIS), for example, the federal government assumed the responsibility and cost of formulating at least the general specifications of an automated system to monitor Medicaid eligibility and use. If the states are given the freedom to implement the various options of beneficiary choice Medicaid, it may be desirable for the federal government to develop the specifications of various prototype health plans. The federal government should also have a role in evaluating and comparing the effectiveness of the programs being implemented at the state level, particularly in the early stages of such a major change in Medicaid, because it will be important to learn what we can from the various state experiences.

The appropriate form of federal-state relationships depends in part on the relative degree of concern voters have for the poor in their own state and the poor in other states and on the flexibility of federal and state bureaucracies. We have suggested qualitative characteristics of some of the more promising mechanisms. Our view is that, once they are in place, superior outcomes will emerge.

Maintaining the Federal-State Partnership

Among recent proposals for dealing with Medicaid are some that would scuttle the federal-state nature of the program entirely, making it a completely federal responsibility. Surprisingly, these proposals have not come from liberal members of the Democratic party, who have long advocated federalized medical care for the poor as part of universal national health insurance. They have come from inside the Reagan administration. In his State of the Union message in 1982, President Reagan proposed full federalization of Medicaid. In return for the federal government's paying the entire cost of Medicaid, the states would accept full responsibility for financing and administering the "cash welfare" programs of Aid to Families with Dependent Children and food stamps. Although the administration has backed off that particular plan, there remains strong interest in somehow dividing up and separating responsibility for the nation's cash and in-kind welfare programs. Placing each type of program in a separate state or federal compartment may reduce the confusion that results from interacting budgetary and regulatory activities, but there are strong reasons to believe that such an attempt at compartmentalization is inferior to alternative reforms for *both* Medicaid and cash welfare.

In general we have argued that the appropriate solution for an overintrusive federal presence in public services jointly financed by states and the national government is not to eliminate cooperative financing; it is rather to substitute indirect control through adjustment of the sharing percentage for direct control through bureaucratic rule making. Our view is that deregulation of Medicaid at the federal level, modification of financing arrangements, and transfer of control to the states are preferable to full federalization.

One of the arguments advanced in favor of complete federal control of both Medicare and Medicaid is that medical costs would somehow be controlled. If this means that the government would exercise monopsony power to pay lower prices for services, the outcome is not necessarily socially efficient, nor is it clear that the federal government would have much more monopsony power in local markets than the states. Alternatively, if the government is not going to behave like a monopsonist, it is unclear why taking over Medicaid will help the federal government do in a politically acceptable way what it has never been able to do with Medicare. There is little evidence that program administrators in the Department of Health and Human Services have somehow found a way to control costs that only they can practice.

If there are no major gains from compartmentalization, however, there could be some major losses. The most serious loss would involve whatever portion of the welfare system is turned over to the states, whether that be AFDC, the long-term-care portion of Medicaid, or other programs that serve low-income people. Even though AFDC is not the main theme of this study, it is worth commenting on this possibility because we have already developed much of the needed background and much of what we have said about federal-state financing arrangements applies to AFDC and other programs as well as to Medicaid.

It is beyond doubt that people care about the levels of welfare benefits (cash and in-kind) in other states as well as their own. The purpose of matching grants in AFDC as in Medicaid was to reflect that concern, by providing an incentive for states to push benefits and eligibility higher than would otherwise have been chosen by state politicians concerned only with the desires of taxpayers in their state. Returning those programs to the state effectively raises the tax price of benefits exactly as discussed in our treatment of block grants for Medicaid. Turning AFDC back to the states would supply an incentive to cut expenditures more than the preferences of taxpayers inside and outside the state, taken together, would indicate; and this incentive to cut program benefits would be stronger for those low-income states that had previously received the largest matching rates. Compensating the states by returning lump-sum excise tax revenues would not help much to offset these incentives, even if the number of dollars were the same, because the incentive would not be the same. In attempting to develop policies that reflect President Reagan's concern about the overintrusive federal presence, strategists in Washington have ignored this simple economic model of human, including political, behavior. Except for those programs—and there are some—in which there is no obvious interest outside a particular state, this is a defect shared by the entire "new federalism" package. If programs are to reflect both the national and the local interests of voters, a truly federal financing system is required for those government activities for which concern crosses state lines.

The proposal to federalize Medicaid fully seems quite inconsistent with the spirit of federalism. Here is a service that is one of the most personal that individuals buy, one that is rendered in very different ways at very different costs in different parts of the country; yet it is proposed that this activity be turned over to the homogenizing influence of the federal bureaucracy. Indeed, if one had to compartmentalize programs, it would be better for the federal government to take over AFDC, since the federal government has shown itself relatively efficient in giving out money and since local circumstances are not likely to have much effect on the technology of writing checks. But better results may be achieved for both Medicaid and AFDC if we simply readjust the sharing percentages, establish some general guidelines, and let the states decide how the money is to be spent, but retain the federal matching to reflect the interest of others in how much is spent.

Another feature of some recent proposals that seems to have little apparent rationale is the plan to split off the long-term-care portion of Medicaid for state administration. We noted above that more than half of Medicaid expenditure goes for the aged and disabled, much of it for custodial care in nursing homes. In many ways, the custodial care benefits of Medicaid are more like income transfers conditioned on the occurrence of serious disability—inability to care for one's self—rather than a payment for medical care per se. If one wants to reshuffle programs (and we do not), it might be more efficient administratively, as well as politically, to combine these maintenance payments with the cash transfer part of social security or SSI. There is already some interaction between these programs; SSI payments are reduced for institutionalized persons, and since many nursing home residents are in a spend-down category, Medicaid needs to know about any income to determine what to pay the nursing home. To be sure, combining what is effectively a health-conditioned welfare program for the aged with social security would harm the illusion that social security is like a private retirement annuity, but this illusion is becoming increasingly transparent as the transfer aspects of the program are becoming more widely recognized.

None of these proposals for dividing the welfare system, including Medicaid, into pieces for separate federal and state administration gets to the heart of the problem. Those who think difficulties with Medicaid and AFDC will somehow go away if administrative responsibilities are reallocated are missing the point; there is little evidence that current problems with the nation's welfare programs derive from the programs' administrative structure. Moreover, unnecessary reorganization can consume scarce management resources, be disruptive to program operations, and sidetrack efforts at more basic reforms. What is really needed is a serious effort to restructure incentives for states, providers, and recipients within the existing federal system

92

so as to promote better use of Medicaid's resources. A corresponding adjustment of federal-state financing arrangements is needed for AFDC as well.

The changes that we recommend would leave the states with the responsibility for administering medical care and cash benefits for the poor of all ages. In our judgment, both cash and medical care programs should receive federal matching funds, but the form of the programs should allow for considerable state discretion—even going so far as to let states substitute cash payments for Medicaid and vice versa, if they so desire.

Improving the Well-Being of the Poor

We have throughout this study simply accepted the objective of cutting Medicaid costs. One is naturally disturbed by actions that reduce poor people's real income, however, and it does no good to pretend that we can somehow separate the truly needy from the undeserving poor. In our view, virtually all Medicaid beneficiaries are needy, although the extent of their need varies. Are there less costly ways to compensate the poor for reductions in Medicaid benefits?

We have already suggested a way in which beneficiaries can turn some of the savings from cutting Medicaid costs into increased cash income for themselves. Consider the following example: A typical four-person Medicaid family (one adult and three children) might have a cash income of about $5,000 and Medicaid insurance with an actuarial value of $2,000. The value of the Medicaid policy constitutes a substantial share of the family's resources. It is quite likely that, given a choice, the family would be willing to give up some of those benefits in return for cash. This might be particularly true if what was given up was mainly the convenience of using nearby providers or amenities in care. If the family prefers cash to benefits in kind, it follows that the minimum amount of cash needed to compensate for a loss in benefits is less than the dollar value of the benefits lost. That is, it would be possible to make the family better off, in its own estimation, by actually spending *less* tax money on it.

The argument here, of course, is the standard economic argument that redistribution in the form of cash is to be preferred to redistribution in kind. Why would it not be better to "cash out" Medicaid? There are, we believe, two arguments against complete cashing out. The first is that the family might choose not to buy insurance coverage and then find itself unable to pay for care during a costly illness. It would be false economy to shift the cost of care for the poor from Medicaid taxes to providers' bad debts, which would have to be covered by revenue from paying patients. It is worth noting that some state Medicaid programs are proposing to do just that in the context of hospital rate regulation. They want the bad debts, whose avoidance is one of Medicaid's purposes, to somehow justify a discount from actual cost for Medicaid. But such a discount, however attractive it may appear to budget-conscious administrators, really only switches the pockets out of which the nonpoor pay the cost of care for the poor—and this amounts to an intellectually dishonest way of moving politically controversial expenditures "off budget."

A second argument against cashing out Medicaid involves the externalities discussed earlier—taxpayers do not want to let recipients spend money as the recipients prefer. One can cloak this interference in terms like regard for "social payoffs" or "minimal level of care," but it ultimately reflects the taxpayers' desire to substitute their own preferences for those of recipients.

Even if these rationales are accepted, however, it is worthwhile to speculate whether they apply to decisions respecting the marginal or last additional Medicaid dollars. Especially if combined with enforcement of laws regarding responsibility—financial responsibility for bills, parental responsibility for the care of children—might it be possible to cash out some Medicaid benefits into positive and more valuable additions to poor people's cash income? What do the marginal dollars of Medicaid really buy? What are they worth to beneficiaries? Would recipients be willing to forgo free choice or dental benefits or complete freedom from copayments in return for larger cash transfers? Answers to these questions might help to pinpoint both the desirability of cuts and the best way to make them, but such information is probably attainable only through further experimentation in the form of either waivered demonstrations or experimental state programs.

Notes

1. Qualified plans under Enthoven's consumer choice health plan would offer at least a basic package of health services with catastrophic expense protection, have annual open enrollment, and use community rating. See Alain Enthoven, *Health Plan* (Reading, Mass.: Addison-Wesley, 1980). A less restrictive definition of health plans has been proposed by Walter McClure, "On Broadening the Definition of and Removing Barriers to a Competitive Health Care System," *Journal of Health Politics, Policy, and Law*, vol. 33 (Fall 1978), pp. 303–27.

2. Joseph P. Newhouse and Vincent Taylor, "A New Type of Hospital Insurance," *Journal of Risk and Insurance*, vol. 38 (December 1971), pp. 601–12.

8

Summary of
Policy Recommendations

In this section we briefly restate some of our more important recommendations for public policy concerning Medicaid. Our major conclusions can be divided into those that relate to federal-state financing arrangements and those that pertain to restructuring incentives for providers and recipients.

In the area of financing, we have examined possible variations ranging from block grants, to a fully national program, to matching-rate schemes. The criteria we selected for evaluating the financing alternatives were recipient equity, taxpayer equity, and satisfaction of voters' preferences. Financing arrangements of two general types would almost certainly fail to achieve those goals and in the end would probably be less politically acceptable than the current federal matching arrangement. These are, first, plans that would reduce federal matching at the margin to zero without ensuring adequate federal or state funding to support benefits at the desired level. Giving states block grants at the current level of federal funding, for example, and allowing them to determine benefits would probably lead them to reduce Medicaid spending to low levels that do not adequately reflect the concern of out-of-state voters. The second type of financing arrangement that is probably best avoided is a wholly national or "federalized" program. We have pointed out a number of problems with a uniform national plan, including the difficulty of structuring benefits to account for differences in local medical care prices and local delivery systems, as well as the need to satisfy the desires of some voters for provision of extra benefits to the poor in their own geographic area. It is also implausible that a homogeneous national program could be the least expensive means of meeting the needs of the poor in the diverse settings in which they are located throughout the United States. In fact, the states appear to have been more effective in controlling the cost of Medicaid than the federal government has been in controlling the cost of Medicare. And there is good reason to let the states continue, although we have suggested how more appropriate incentives and fewer federal restrictions could aid states in their cost-controlling efforts. What is needed is a deliberate decision to avoid direct federal control, including unnecessary strings on federal dollars, and to let fiscal incentives inherent in appropriate federal matching do their job.

The type of financing arrangement that we favor would allow for state administration with continued federal financial support. We have identified two particularly attractive mechanisms. One would make matching rates a decreasing function of state expenditures. Such rates would be determined by the number of poor people in the state, local medical care prices, and the state's aggregate taxpayer income or tax base. States would receive the most federal assistance (perhaps 100 percent) for bringing benefits up to some national minimum, but they would have to pay an increasing share of the cost as benefits per poor person were expanded above the U.S. average. A lump-sum state contribution to the program might be used to equalize tax burdens. An alternative arrangement would combine a federal block grant with a requirement that each state contribute enough funds to meet a national minimum standard of real benefits. The state could expand benefits beyond this point if it wished, perhaps with some federal assistance. Either of these arrangements, if properly designed and implemented, would lead to more uniform real Medicaid expenditures per poor person and more uniform tax burdens among the states.

We have also considered a number of possible means of altering incentives for providers and Medicaid recipients. We have focused on means of limiting medical care use per recipient because this has been the source of much of the recent growth in real (inflation-adjusted) Medicaid spending. In general, we have favored those alternatives that give recipients the most freedom to determine their own patterns of use but with incentives for them to select less costly providers and to avoid using services that have a low value in relation to their costs.

Many mechanisms for making beneficiaries and providers more sensitive to costs have recently been discussed in connection with various proposals to promote competition in the medical care sector. Features such as copayments, HMOs, and health plans can—when adapted to the special needs of the people Medicaid serves—lead to cost savings that will allow states to reduce expenditures or expand eligibility. We have also noted how limits on reimbursement rates and prudent buyer arrangements save costs, at the expense of reducing the access of beneficiaries to some providers. The adverse effect of such policies on freedom to choose the most preferred provider could be reduced (at no increase in public cost) by allowing recipients to supplement public reimbursement with payments out of their own pockets. Our most preferred form of Medicaid would offer beneficiaries a choice among several competing plans, ranging from full-coverage insurance, to HMO-type health plans, to various cost-sharing arrangements.

In this monograph we have developed some guidelines for future Medicaid policy involving federal-state financing and administration, competitive incentives for providers, and considerable choice for recipients. Full implementation of such policies obviously will require more information than is now available on responses of states, providers, and recipients to proposed changes. Understandably, policy makers will be reluctant to adopt major program changes without some certainty about where they will lead. Nevertheless, we believe that enough information is available to begin making the changes we propose. Policies may be implemented gradually, and plans can be modified as states experiment and as new information becomes available from demonstrations and evaluations. Achieving some degree of consensus on where the Medicaid program should be heading, however, is a precondition for that process.

Appendix A

Demand for Transfers in a Federal System

The theory of public goods provides a basis for determining a socially optimal level of provision for jointly consumed commodities. This theory can be applied to Medicaid. Medical care for the poor can be considered a public good, in that the benefits of knowing that the poor have adequate medical care accrue freely to everyone without the possibility of exclusion. Medicaid therefore has the properties of nonrivalness in consumption and nonexcludability that characterize public goods. The theory of redistribution as a public good has been dealt with in a number of previous studies, including some that deal specifically with transfers in kind.[1] These models have also been cast in a public choice framework and used to explain programs such as AFDC, food stamps, and Medicaid.[2] These applications employ the concept of a representative or median voter to explain government expenditures.

A criterion for efficient provision of a public good is that the sum of the marginal valuations of all affected persons be equal to the marginal cost of the goods. As described less technically in the text, this condition requires that the public good be produced at the point where the vertical summation of individual demand curves intersects the marginal cost curve.

A simplified example may be useful in illustrating some of the relationships between factors that determine the provision of Medicaid benefits in a federal system. Consider a nation consisting of two states identical except that the income of state taxpayers is higher in one of the states than in the other. The states are assumed (for now) to have the same number of poor people and identical prices. Taxpayers are assumed to be equally concerned about consumption of medical care by the poor regardless of where the poor reside. That is, preferences for redistribution are not local.

The differences in Medicaid expenditures resulting from differences in state income are represented in figure A-1. The D_L and D_H curves respectively represent the hypothetical in-state demand of a

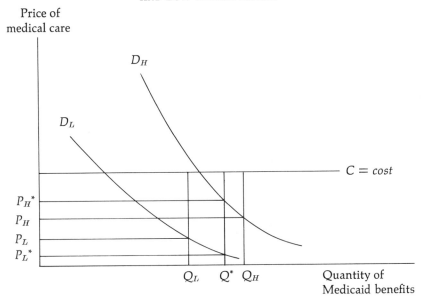

low-income and a high-income state for Medicaid. The high-income
state receives a 50 percent subsidy on Medicaid benefits and therefore
pays an effective price of $(1 - 0.5)C$, shown as P_H in the figure.[3] This
subsidy induces the state to select an aggregate quantity of real
benefits of Q_H, a much greater quantity than that chosen by the low-
income state, Q_L, even though the low-income state faces a low effective price, P_L, because of its higher matching rate. The optimal quantity
of Medicaid benefits is the same in each of the states since they are
identical except for taxpayers' income. The optimum quantity, Q^*,
may be greater or less than Q_H, but it must be to the right of the
point where the demand curve, D_H, crosses the marginal cost curve.
This is because the sum of marginal valuations of all states must
be at least as great as the marginal valuation in the state with the
greatest demand. In this example, the high-income state could be
induced to reduce its benefits to the optimal quantity by lowering its
matching rate until the effective price of providing additional benefits
was raised to P_H^* Similarly, a greater matching rate leading to price
P_L^* would induce the low-income state to provide the optimal quantity
of benefits.

The figure shows that it is possible to find matching rates that satisfy both (1) recipient equity—in the sense that the quantity of medical care provided per poor person is the same in each state—and (2) the satisfaction of voters' demand, since the optimum, Q^*, is achieved and both states provide benefits according to their demand curves given the appropriate matching rates. The issue of taxpayer equity is in doubt, however, and an assessment of this condition requires additional information on taxpayers' income that is not reflected in the figure. A more formal analysis is called for.

Consider the following conditions, which are defined in terms of a fifty-state nation in which each state's spending is matched by the federal government at a constant rate.

Recipient Equity (RE). The recipient equity condition can be expressed as

$$Q_S/N_S = K^* \qquad S = 1, \ldots, 50 \qquad (1)$$

where Q_S is the aggregate quantity of benefits in state S, N_S is the number of poor people, and K^* is the optimal benefit per poor person. In this simple example, K^* is the same in every state. The recipient equity condition thus requires that Medicaid payments per poor person in real terms (adjusted for price differences) be the same in every state.

Taxpayer Equity (TE). The taxpayer equity condition can be expressed as

$$Q_S C_S(1 - F_S) = t^* Y_S \qquad S = 1, \ldots, 50 \qquad (2)$$

where C_S is the local cost of medical services, F_S is the federal matching share in state S, Y_S is the state's aggregate taxpayer income, and t^* is the voters' tax share for state Medicaid expenditures. The condition requires that the state's contribution to Medicaid as a share of aggregate taxpayer income be the same in each state.

Demand Satisfaction (DS). The voter demand satisfaction condition can be expressed as

$$Q_S = D_S[Y_S, (1 - F_S) \ C_S, N_S] \qquad S = 1, \ldots, 50 \qquad (3)$$

where D_S is a state demand function with the following arguments: taxpayers' income, after-matching price to the state of providing medical benefits, and the number of poor people in the state.

As expressed, RE and TE are weak conditions in that they do not require that every poor person be provided exactly the same benefits or that every taxpayer have exactly the same tax burden. The conditions only require that the average benefit or burden be the same in every state. The precise distribution of benefits and tax burden could depend on the state's Medicaid program and tax structure. Despite the fact that the conditions are relatively weak, however, they are sufficiently constraining to be mutually exclusive, at least in the case of simple matching rates.

> PROPOSITION: *It is not generally possible to find a set of matching rates that will satisfy RE, TE, and DS simultaneously.*

For the fifty-state nation we have a system of 150 equations with 101 undetermined variables—50 Q's, 50 F's, and t^* (K^* is determined by the selection of the optimal benefit per poor person). Because the number of undetermined variables is less than the number of relations to be satisfied, the equations will be inconsistent except in special cases. That is, there is no set of matching rates that will satisfy RE, TE, and DS. This result points out the futility of even attempting to manipulate simple matching rates to achieve recipient and taxpayer equity while allowing states to determine their own benefit levels.

Adding a Lump-Sum State Contribution. The inconsistency of the three goals RE, TE, and DS derives from an insufficient number of undetermined variables in the system of equations representing these three conditions. If, however, we allow for the possibility of an additional lump-sum payment (positive or negative) between the state and federal governments, then tax burdens among states can be equalized. The taxpayer equity condition becomes

$$Q_S C_S (1 - F_S) + L_S = t^* Y_S \qquad S = 1, \ldots, 50 \qquad (4)$$

where L_S is the lump-sum payment. With the RE and DS equations for each of fifty states, we have a system of 150 equations and 151 undetermined variables including the L's and the tax burden, t^*. With well-behaved and known demand functions, it is then possible to solve for a set of matching rates and lump-sum payments that satisfy RE, TE, and DS. Proceed by simultaneously solving equations (1) and (3) for matching rates designed to provide RE and DS. These rates, denoted F_S^{**}, will induce states to set benefits at an optimal level. Then the required lump-sum payment is

$$L_S = t^* Y_S - K^* N_S C_S (1 - F_S^{**}) \qquad S = 1, \ldots, 50$$

It then remains to ensure that the lump sum required of the state is not so large as to cause the state to opt out of the Medicaid program altogether. Figure A-2 shows state and total (internal plus external)

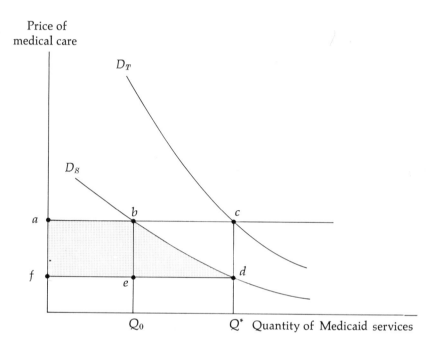

FIGURE A-2
MAXIMUM LUMP-SUM STATE CONTRIBUTION TO MEDICAID

demand for Medicaid within a particular state. With the optimal matching rate, F_s^{**}, the state would choose to provide Q^* units of Medicaid benefits. Note that in the absence of subsidy the state would choose to provide benefits at Q_0. To determine the size of lump-sum contributions the state is willing to pay to participate, we compare the consumer surplus the state derives from participation with the added cost. By participating in the program, the state increases aggregate Medicaid benefits by $Q^* - Q_0$ units and adds the area enclosed by *abdf* to its consumer surplus. This area represents the amount the state would be willing to pay to participate. Note that this is at least as great as the federal share of the quantity the state would provide without federal assistance, but something less than the federal government would spend in matching payments alone at Q^*.

Block Grants with State Contributions. It is possible to set the block grants and state contributions at levels that would promote both recipient and taxpayer equity. The federal government must choose the desired (preferably optimal) level of benefits per poor person, K^*, and the tax rate, t^*, that taxpayers must pay for Medicaid through state taxes. Then we can calculate the size of the federal block grant to each state and the size of each state's lump-sum contribution. These are, respectively,

$$G_S = K^* N_S C_S - t^* Y_S \qquad S = 1, \ldots, 50$$
$$L_S = t^* Y_S \qquad S = 1, \ldots, 50$$

where Y_S is aggregate taxpayer income in the state, C is an index of medical care prices in the state, and N is the number of persons below the poverty level in that state. With grants and state contributions set in this manner, the state tax burden (as a fraction of income) would be the same for the typical taxpayer in all states, and the total funds available to the Medicaid program would permit delivery of the same quantity of real benefits per poor person in each state. The value of t^* must be sufficiently low (and thus L sufficiently small) that states do not choose to drop out of the program. The maximum feasible state contribution is determined with the consumer surplus approach described above.

Notes

1. See Harold M. Hochman and James D. Rodgers, "Pareto Optimal Redistribution," *American Economic Review*, vol. 59 (1969), pp. 542–59; George M. von Furstenberg and Dennis C. Mueller, "The Pareto Optimal Approach to Income Redistribution: A Fiscal Approach," *American Economic Review* (September 1971); Edgar K. Browning, "A Comment on Distributional Externalities and In-Kind Transfers," *Public Finance Quarterly* (1976); idem, "The Diagrammatic Analysis of Multiple Consumption Externalities," *American Economic Review*, vol. 64 (September 1974), pp. 707–14; and Edgar O. Olson, "Some Theorems in the Theory of Efficient Transfers," *Journal of Political Economy* (January–February 1971), pp. 166–75.

2. See Larry L. Orr, "Income Transfers as a Public Good: An Application to AFDC," *American Economic Review*, vol. 66 (June 1976), pp. 19–35; Thomas Grannemann, "The Demand for Publicly Financed Medical Care: The Role of Interdependent Preferences" (Ph.D. dissertation, Northwestern University, 1979); J. Fred Giertz and Dennis H. Sullivan, "Donor Optimization and the Food Stamp Program," *Public Choice*, vol. 32 (Spring 1977), pp. 19–35.

3. We ignore the effect that changes in a particular state's Medicaid benefits will have on the state's taxpayers' federal taxes. This effect is small; so we treat the state's effective price as simply the state share times the marginal cost.

Appendix B

Beneficiary Choice Medicaid: An Example

In this appendix we outline the basic features of a possible "beneficiary choice" Medicaid program. The fundamental proposition is that responsibility for controlling Medicaid costs and the power to do so should be transferred from the federal government to the states and from the states to individual beneficiaries and providers. Beneficiary choice arrangements would

- abolish all federal requirements for state Medicaid benefit packages except some upper limits on out-of-pocket expense as a percentage of beneficiaries' income
- encourage the states to offer voucher-like arrangements to beneficiaries
- alter the current form of federal-state financing so that the matching rate is an increasing function of the number of poor people in the state and of medical care prices and a decreasing function of total taxpayers' income in the state (or some other measure of fiscal capacity), with the objective of producing more nearly equal expenditures per poor person (the arrangement might require states to contribute a lump sum to the program in an amount that would tend to equalize tax burdens among states)[1]

The plans for the beneficiary to choose from would be of three types:

Type 1: State-administered and -determined state Medicaid plan (SMP)
  a. Plan would be available to all beneficiaries at no direct cost.
  b. Plan would be similar to current Medicaid, at least initially, with low or zero copayments and free choice of providers.
  c. Plan's average cost would determine the actuarial value of benefit (AVB) for each category, as defined by age,

sex, location, chronic conditions (actual classifying variables would have to be determined).

    d. Plan would be publicly produced.

Type 2: Full coverage plan (FCP)

    a. Plan would have same nominal coverage as SMP, but with limits on choice of provider. It would include HMOs, health care alliances, and plans with limits of participating physicians and hospitals. At a minimum it would cover all services included in the state Medicaid plan (SMP).

    b. Plan would be privately produced.

    c. Plan would determine actuarial cost for the set of benefits offered by SMP, called basic premium (BP).

    d. State would establish cost-saving percentage, between 1 and 99 percent, denoted C.

    e. Beneficiary unit that selected FCP would receive a bonus of $C(AVB - BP)$. If premium for an FCP were greater than AVB, the beneficiary could still use the plan by paying the difference.

Type 3: Cost-sharing plans (CSP)

    a. Privately operated insurance plans would offer insurance with cost sharing. Both the maximum cost-sharing percentage and the maximum share of family income devoted to cost sharing would be subject to state limits.

    b. The private insurers could accept vouchers as payment for the insurance, and the state could maintain its own insurance plans as well.

    c. The bonus would consist of two parts. The first part would be the difference between the AVB amount and the total expected cost of medical care for the family. That is, it would equal $(AVB - PRE - ACS)$, where PRE is the premium and ACS is the actuarial value of the cost sharing. The second part of the bonus would consist of the difference (positive or negative) between the actuarial value of cost sharing and the actual cost-sharing amount the family had incurred. This means that if a family selected a plan with cost sharing that did not reduce its expected total expenditures below those of the state plan, the first part of its bonus would be zero, and the second part would of course have an expected value of zero. Hence it would expect zero gain. In contrast, if it selected a plan associated with lower total medical care costs, its expected gain would be C times the amount of the first part of the bonus. Adding an income limit on total expenses would make the calculations more complex but would not change the basic idea.

Examples of Four Options

Consider a four-person beneficiary family with expected covered expenses under SMP of $3,000. Suppose the state sets the cost-sharing percentage (C) at 60 percent. The family's choices might be as follows:

Option 1: state medical plan. No premium would be required, and no bonus would be paid.

Option 2: full coverage plan. Under this option the family would use an HMO that had contracted with the state to provide services to Medicaid clients at a negotiated rate. The HMO would have the same service coverage as the state plan and a contract price of $2,700. The family would receive a bonus of 60 percent of the cost saving, or $180; the state would pay $120 less in Medicaid costs.

Option 3: augmented full coverage plan. This plan would provide additional dental coverage as well as basic benefits. The HMO would have an expected cost of $2,650 for the basic benefits but charge $2,750 for the expanded package. The family could use its voucher to cover the cost and, in addition, would receive a bonus of $110. In effect, part of the bonus would be applied to the cost of extra benefits.

Option 4: cost-sharing plan. For simplicity, we discuss a plan with no income-conditioned limits on total expenditures. The plan might offer insurance with a copayment per physician visit of $10. The actuarial value of these out-of-pocket payments would be $150 and the premium for the insurance $2,650. The first part of the bonus would therefore be 0.6 ($3,000-$2,650-$150), or $120. The maximum value the second part of the bonus could take would be $150; so the gross bonus would be $270, and this amount would be received by a family that made no visits to a physician in a year. If it made ten visits, its bonus would be $170, and if it made twenty visits (an above-average amount), its bonus would be $70. Of course, if it made the average number of visits, fifteen, its net bonus would be $120, just equal to its share of the expected savings from choosing this insurance. The state would gain an average of $80 for each family that chose this program.

Note

1. As an alternative to changing matching rates, one could provide block grants to states with mandatory state contributions. Grants could be designed to make resources available to each state to allow for equal real benefits per poor person, to set state contributions to equalize tax burdens among states, and to permit states to supplement the minimum amount at their own expense.

Appendix C

Tables and Data Sources

This appendix lists the sources of the data employed in the computer simulation of chapter 5 and presents data by state in Tables C-1 and C-2 here.

Data Sources

1. Medicaid medical vendor payments and numbers of Medicaid recipients—Medicaid State Tables for Fiscal Year 1980, revised final February 1, 1982, prepublished, Medicaid Program Data Branch, Office of Research, Health Care Financing Administration.

2. Federal medical assistance percentages—*Federal Register,* December 1, 1980, p. 79582.

3. Personal income per capita, 1981, and average hourly earnings for production workers (for price index)—U.S. Bureau of the Census, *Statistical Abstract of the United States, 1981,* 102d ed. (Washington, D.C., December 1981).

4. Number of persons below the poverty level—U.S. Bureau of the Census, *1980 Census of Population and Housing Supplementary Report Provisional Estimates of Social, Economic, and Housing Characteristics* (Washington, D.C., March 1982).

5. Adjusted gross income of taxpayers—U.S. Internal Revenue Service, *Statistics of Income Bulletin* (Winter 1981–1982).

6. Hospital cost per patient-day (for price index)—Health Insurance Association of America, *Source Book of Health Insurance Data 1981–1982* (Washington, D.C.).

7. Physician specialist fee index (for price index)—Ira Burney et al., "Geographic Variation in Physicians' Fees," *Journal of the American Medical Association* (September 22, 1978), pp. 1368–71.

TABLE C–1

	Recipients as Percentage of Poor Population	Medicaid Payments per Poor Person	Real Benefits per Poor Person	Medical Care Price Index	State Medicaid Expenditures as Percentage of Taxpayers' Income
Northeast					
Connecticut	83	1,335	1,233	108	0.62
Maine	104	938	1,073	87	0.61
Massachusetts	142	1,847	1,619	114	1.09
New Hampshire	58	923	1,099	84	0.43
New Jersey	97	1,081	1,173	92	0.60
New York	98	1,938	1,779	109	1.74
Pennsylvania	103	872	909	96	0.57
Rhode Island	136	1,711	1,665	103	1.06
Vermont	97	1,065	1,376	77	0.61
South					
Alabama	47	385	434	89	0.36
Arkansas	53	562	709	79	0.58
Delaware	72	660	681	97	0.49
District of Columbia	110	1,465	1,068	137	1.52
Florida	40	315	309	102	0.25
Georgia	49	532	588	91	0.47
Kentucky	62	450	569	79	0.48
Louisiana	47	534	560	95	0.52
Maryland	76	781	766	102	0.47
Mississippi	51	352	480	73	0.40
North Carolina	46	485	613	79	0.38
Oklahoma	65	679	699	97	0.54
South Carolina	70	541	686	79	0.44
Tennessee	47	499	588	85	0.45
Texas	33	477	510	94	0.42
Virginia	54	604	699	86	0.40
West Virginia	47	375	458	82	0.31
North-Central					
Illinois	82	928	840	110	0.66
Indiana	39	678	767	88	0.41
Iowa	67	865	1,028	84	0.52
Kansas	64	871	1,011	86	0.57
Michigan	97	1,067	1,007	106	0.81

(Table continues)

TABLE C–1 (continued)

	Recipients as Percentage of Poor Population	Medicaid Payments per Poor Person	Real Benefits per Poor Person	Medical Care Price Index	State Medicaid Expenditures as Percentage of Taxpayers' Income
Minnesota	88	1,598	1,883	85	0.91
Missouri	54	498	533	93	0.36
Nebraska	45	686	843	81	0.43
North Dakota	39	585	774	76	0.44
Ohio	73	730	750	97	0.48
South Dakota	33	513	650	79	0.47
Wisconsin	109	1,767	1,967	90	0.88
West					
Alaska	44	682	438	156	0.33
California	103	1,045	753	139	0.72
Colorado	49	629	639	99	0.38
Hawaii	116	1,045	1,055	99	0.66
Idaho	37	441	510	87	0.33
Montana	48	656	900	73	0.43
Nevada	38	670	500	134	0.33
New Mexico	40	316	308	102	0.30
Oregon	95	615	565	109	0.45
Utah	37	518	492	105	0.29
Washington	77	803	761	105	0.50
Wyoming	30	393	408	96	0.18
United States[a]	73	847	847	100	0.66

a. U.S. averages exclude Puerto Rico and Virgin Islands. Arizona did not have a Medicaid program in 1980.
Source: Calculated using data from the sources listed in this appendix.

TABLE C–2

MEDICAID PAYMENTS PER RECIPIENT, BY ELIGIBILITY CATEGORY AND
BY STATE, FISCAL YEAR 1980

(dollars)

	Medicaid Payments per Elderly Recipient	Medicaid Payments per Child Recipient	Medicaid Payments per Adult Recipient
Northeast			
Connecticut	4,729	466	787
Maine	779	561	1,059
Massachusetts	3,025	280	777
New Hampshire	4,616	215	965
New Jersey	4,447	334	676
New York	6,015	610	1,158
Pennsylvania	2,870	286	438
Rhode Island	3,100	261	539
Vermont	2,630	304	520
South			
Alabama	1,360	239	589
Arkansas	1,575	273	642
Delaware	3,120	288	632
District of Columbia	3,122	562	1,154
Florida	1,465	258	540
Georgia	1,672	272	1,004
Kentucky	1,295	240	549
Louisiana	1,760	358	651
Maryland	2,885	460	810
Mississippi	1,253	238	488
North Carolina	1,971	265	685
Oklahoma	2,120	357	516
South Carolina	1,556	171	528
Tennessee	1,757	353	702
Texas	2,008	283	847
Virginia	2,325	296	677
West Virginia	1,457	365	595
North-Central			
Illinois	2,971	426	967
Indiana	4,447	259	782
Iowa	2,910	330	692
Kansas	3,099	413	759

(Table continues)

TABLE C–2 (continued)

	Medicaid Payments per Elderly Recipient	Medicaid Payments per Child Recipient	Medicaid Payments per Adult Recipient
Michigan	2,947	349	950
Minnesota	5,060	320	504
Missouri	1,782	283	641
Nebraska	3,086	376	733
North Dakota	3,473	405	804
Ohio	2,151	300	695
South Dakota	3,180	297	675
Wisconsin	4,212	440	735
West			
Alaska	4,009	437	662
California	1,319	316	684
Colorado	2,292	246	642
Hawaii	3,027	328	772
Idaho	2,890	300	613
Montana	3,638	257	709
Nevada	3,020	367	854
New Mexico	1,519	275	655
Oregon	1,719	158	401
Utah	3,298	225	593
Washington	2,703	288	635
Wyoming	3,832	342	859
United States[a]	2,544	355	748

a. U.S. averages exclude Puerto Rico and Virgin Islands. Arizona did not have a Medicaid program in this period.
SOURCE: Calculated using data from the sources listed in this appendix.

SELECTED AEI PUBLICATIONS

Passing the Health Care Buck: Who Pays the Hidden Cost? Jack A. Meyer, with William R. Johnson and Sean Sullivan (49 pp., $3.95)

Competition in the Pharmaceutical Industry: The Declining Profitability of Drug Innovation, Meir Statman (84 pp., $4.95)

Economics and Medical Research, Burton A. Weisbrod (171 pp., cloth $15.95, paper $7.95)

Market Reforms in Health Care: Current Issues, New Directions, Strategic Decisions, Jack A. Meyer, ed. (331 pp., cloth $19.95, paper $10.95)

Meeting Human Needs: Toward a New Public Philosophy, Jack A. Meyer, ed. (469 pp., cloth $34.95, paper $13.95)

Medicaid Reimbursement of Nursing-Home Care, Paul L. Grimaldi (194 pp., cloth $15.95, paper $7.95)

A New Approach to the Economics of Health Care, Mancur Olson, ed. (502 pp., cloth $18.25, paper $10.25)

Drugs and Health: Economic Issues and Policy Objectives, Robert B. Helms, ed. (344 pp., cloth $16.25, paper $8.25)

International Supply of Medicines: Implications of U.S. Regulatory Reform, Robert B. Helms, ed. (156 pp., cloth $14.25, paper $6.25)

Tropical Diseases: Responses of Pharmaceutical Companies, Jack N. Behrman (80 pp., $4.25)

National Health Insurance: What Now, What Later, What Never?, Mark V. Pauly, ed. (381 pp., cloth $16.25, paper $8.25)

National Health Insurance in Ontario: The Effects of a Policy of Cost Control, William S. Comanor (57 pp., $4.25)

National Health Insurance: Now, Later, Never? John Charles Daly, mod. (25 pp., $3.75)

Prices subject to change without notice.

• *Mail orders for publications to:* AMERICAN ENTERPRISE INSTITUTE, 1150 Seventeenth Street, N.W., Washington, D.C. 20036 • *For postage and handling, add 10 percent of total; minimum charge, $2* • *For information on orders, or to expedite service, call toll free* 800-424-2873 • *Prices subject to change without notice.* • *Payable in U.S. currency only.*